规范体格检查与病史书写双语手册

Physical examination and case history-bilingual learning handbook

主编 傅志君 石 虹
　　　Fu Zhijun　Shi　Hong

复旦大学出版社

主编	傅志君 Fu Zhijun	石 虹 Shi Hong		
编者	(按姓氏笔画排序)			
	石 虹 Shi Hong	朱文青 Zhu Wenqing	王葆青 Wang Baoqing	叶志斌 Ye Zhibin
	钟春玖 Zhong Chunjiu	傅志君 Fu Zhijun	严震文 Yan Zhenwen	林豪杰 Lin Haojie
	赖雁妮 Lai Yanni	徐蓓莉 Xu Beili		

前　言

为了帮助医学生掌握病史书写和体格检查的基本内容和正确手法，并结合八年制双语教学改革的要求，我们按照脏器系统顺序进行排列，编写了《规范体格检查与病史书写双语手册》。

体格检查是医生用自己的感官或借助传统的辅助工具对病人进行全面检查，找出机体正常或异常的征象，这是诊断疾病最客观的证据之一。检查正确与否，直接关系到能否对病人作出正确的诊断和治疗。因此，体格检查和病史书写是诊断学教学的重要内容，是各科临床医师必须掌握的基本功。

按脏器系统顺序对医学生进行全身体格检查训练，比较容易掌握。为了减少病人的体位变动，在反复练习、熟练掌握全身体格检查的技能后，可打破脏器系统顺序，按照身体大的部位进行体格检查，即在一般状态检查后，按头部—颈部—前胸部—后胸部—腹部—四肢—肛门、直肠和生殖器排序，而淋巴结、血管、神经系统的检查可穿插在各个部位的检查之中。

本手册附中英文住院病史范例，供医学生书写病史时参阅。

感谢所有编者的辛勤劳动，感谢 Rajina Thakali 同学为本手册的编写提供了很多宝贵的意见。

　　本手册是《诊断学》的辅助教材,希望对广大医学生的学习有所帮助。由于编者水平所限,难免有不妥之处,希望读者批评指正。

傅志君

2009年5月

Preface

In order that the medical students can learn easily the correct technique and the general content, we compile this *manual*, in the order of organs and systems.

Physical check-up is a thorough examination for patients. By using their proper sensors or some traditional tools, doctors can find different symptoms of the patients, normal or abnormal. This is one of the most objective evidence for diagnosing a disease. The correctness of the check-up can direct the diagnosis and the treatment later. So physical check-up is an important content of the diagnostics, it is also a basic skill that must be mastered by a clinician of all specialties.

It is easy to manage if we train the students in the systems' order. But for the patients' convenience, we should change their posture much less if possible. After practice again and again, and well master the skill of check-up, we can broke the order of organs and systems, then examine the patient part after part. That is to say, after the general examination, we check the human body in this order: head-neck-chest-back-abdomen-extremity-anus-rectum-genitalia, the check of lymph nodes, blood vessels and nerves can be included in the whole process.

Finally, we would like to express our gratitude to all the authors for their hard work. We would also like to thank Rajina Thakali for her suggestions. We appreciate all the comments and corrections from the readers. This will help us to improve the next edition.

Fu Zhijun(傅志君)
May, 2009

目 录

第一章　体格检查的准备工作 …………… 1
Chapter 1　General Preparation ………… 2
第二章　一般状态检查 …………………… 3
Chapter 2　General Examination ………… 5
第三章　淋巴结、头颈部检查 …………… 8
Chapter 3　Head, Neck and Lymph
　　　　　　Nodes Exam ………………… 14
第四章　胸廓、肺部检查 ………………… 23
Chapter 4　Examination of Thorax and Lung
　　　　　　……………………………… 26
第五章　心脏、血管检查 ………………… 32
Chapter 5　Cardiovascular Examination …… 34
第六章　腹部检查 ………………………… 38
Chapter 6　Abdominal Examination ……… 44
第七章　脊柱、四肢、神经反射检查 …… 53
Chapter 7　Examinations of Spine,
　　　　　　Extremities and Nervous System
　　　　　　……………………………… 57
第八章　肛门、直肠、生殖器检查 ……… 64
Chapter 8　Examination of Rectum, Anus
　　　　　　and Genitalia ………………… 65
第九章　住院病史 ………………………… 67
Chapter 9　Complete History …………… 73

第一节　住院病史-1 …………… 67
Complete History-1 ……………… 73
第二节　住院病史-2 …………… 81
Complete History-2 ……………… 87

附录1 《规范体格检查及病史书写双语手册》中文—英文单词表………… 95

附录2 《规范体格检查及病史书写双语手册》英文—中文单词表 ………… 104

附录3 《临床诊断学》中文—英文单词表……………………………… 113

附录4 《临床诊断学》英文—中文单词表……………………………… 141

第一章 体格检查的准备工作

1. 体格检查的常用器具包括体温表、血压计、听诊器、叩诊锤、软尺、直尺、手电筒、消毒棉签、压舌板、标记笔等。

2. 医生要仪表端庄、举止大方。检查时要尊重病人、态度和蔼,应先自我介绍,礼貌用语。注意保护病人隐私。

3. 检查的房间应有充足的自然光,以及安静和温暖的环境。

4. 重危病人因病情严重,不允许做详细的体格检查时,则应根据主要临床表现,在进行重点的体格检查后,立即进行抢救治疗,待病情好转后,再做必要的补充检查。

(傅志君)

Chapter 1   General Preparation

1. The equipments needed for physical examination include: clinical thermometer, sphygmomanometer, stethoscope, plexor, ruler, flashlight, disinfectant cotton swabs, spatula, marking pen, et al.

2. Examiner needs to be properly dressed and should have a decent behavior. He/She must respect the patients and protect their privacy. Before proceeding the P. E. must introduce himself/herself to the patient with courtesy and take permission for proceeding the examination.

3. The examination room must have enough sunlight or well lit, should be quiet and warm.

4. Patients in need of intensive care, need to have urgent and appropriate P. E. relevant to the symptoms and the medication. The examiner could proceed the rest of the assisting physical examination only after the patients' condition turns stable.

Lai Yanni(赖雁妮)

第二章 一般状态检查

取体温表,先检查体温表内水银柱是否已甩至35℃以下,然后把体温表放在左腋窝深处紧贴皮肤,如有汗液则必须擦干后测体温,并嘱被检查者用上臂将体温表夹紧,放置约10分钟。

检查脉搏时手指并拢,以示指、中指和环指的指腹平放在被检查者右手桡动脉近手腕处,至少计数30秒(有明显脉律不齐时,需计数1分钟)脉搏搏动的次数。同时观察病人呼吸,计算胸廓起伏频率,计数呼吸频率次数至少30秒。

测量右上臂血压前必须在安静环境下休息5~10分钟。先打开血压计开关,检查水银柱液面是否与0点平齐。测压时被检查者右上肢应裸露、伸直并外展约45°,袖带气囊胶管避开肱动脉,袖带紧贴皮肤缚于上臂,下缘距肘弯横纹约2~3 cm;袖带不宜过紧或过松,一般以能伸进1指为宜。在肘窝肱二头肌肌腱内侧触及肱动脉,将听诊器膜型体件置于肱动脉上,不宜将体件塞在袖带下,卧位时使测量点与腋中线同一水平(坐位时测量点宜置于右心房水平,相当于第4肋软骨)。右手以均匀节奏向气袖内注气,待动脉搏动消失,汞柱再升高20~30 mmHg(2.6~4.0 kPa)。然后缓缓放气,使水银柱以每秒2 mm速度缓慢下降。两眼平视水银柱平面,听到第一次搏动声为收缩压，水银柱继续下降至声音突然变低沉，直至消失，此消失时所示压力值为舒张压。同样的方法测定两次，两次间歇 1 分钟左右，取最低值为血压值。解下袖带，整理好后放入血压计内。向右侧倾斜血压计约 45°，使水银柱内水银进入水银槽内后，关闭血压计开关。

取出体温表，分别记录每分钟脉搏和呼吸的次数、血压和体温。

观察被检查者发育、营养、体型、面容表情和体位。

观察皮肤黏膜有无苍白、发绀、黄染、色素沉着、皮疹、出血点、水肿、肝掌、蜘蛛痣等，并观察毛发分布的情况，检查上臂内侧肘上 3～4 cm 处皮肤弹性。检查前臂曲侧脂肪充实程度。

（傅志君）

Chapter 2　General Examination

Take a clinical thermometer, ensure that the mercury reading is under 35℃. Put the clinical thermometer in the deep of left armpit and closely attached to the skin. The sweats should be wiped off before taking the reading. The patient should be told to seat stable with its upper arm closed for about 10 minutes.

Take the pulse putting the tips of your index, middle and ring fingers over the right radial artery for at least 30 seconds. Count for 30 seconds and multiplied by 2. If the rhythm is irregular the pulse must be repeatedly checked for 1 minute. At the same time count the respiratory rate, the undulation of thoracic cage.

Keep the examinee rest for 5 ~ 10 minutes before you take the blood pressure of right upper arm. Switch on the sphygmomanometer and ensure the mercury level is horizontal with the zero point. Bare the right upper arm and keep the position of stretch and extend about 45 degrees. Affix the collapsed cuff close to the arm, the lower edge lies 2 ~ 3 cm above the elbow and keep the pipe away from the brachial artery. The tightness of cuff should be moderate, and it is better that you can put one finger into it. Palpate for the exact location of the brachial arterial pulse in the biceps-triceps furrow tendon. Put the bell of the stethoscope on the brachial artery and avoid putting the bell inside the cuff. Keep the sphygmomanometer at the level of the fore auxiliary line. Inflate the cuff to a pressure about 20 ~ 30 mmHg above the point where the palpable pulse disappears. Open the valve slightly so the pressure drops gradually at the speed of 2 mm per second. Note the pressure reading at which sound first become audible. This reading is taken as the systolic pressure. As the deflation proceeds, the sound become muffled, take the reading at the point where the sound disappeared as the diastolic pressure. Measure at least two times with the interval of 1 minute and take the lowest reading as the blood pressure. Take off the cuff, clean up and put it back to the sphygmomanometer. Incline the sphygmomanometer right about 45 degrees to keep the mercury into the trough and then switch off the valve.

Take out the thermometer record the pulse rate, respiratory rate, blood pressure and temperature. These are the vital signs.

Inspect the growth, nutrition, shape, facial expression and position of the examinee.

Inspect the skin for pallor, cyanosis, stained yellow, pigmentation, eruption, petechia, edema, liver palm, spider angioma, et al. Notice the distribution of the hair. Examine the flexibility of the skin in the interior of upper arm, 3 ~ 4 cm above the elbow. Examine the fat distribution in the flexible flank of forearms.

Lai Yanni(赖雁妮)

第三章 淋巴结、头颈部检查

浅表淋巴结按顺序由浅入深用双手并拢的示、中、环指的指腹进行滑动触诊,触诊部位有耳周淋巴结群(耳前、耳后、乳头区、枕骨下区),颈深淋巴结上群,颈深淋巴结下群,颌下淋巴结,颏下淋巴结,锁骨上淋巴结(位于锁骨与胸锁乳突肌所形成的夹角处),腋窝淋巴结群,滑车上淋巴结,腹股沟淋巴结群,腘窝淋巴结。应注意淋巴结肿大的部位、大小、数目、质地、压痛、活动度、有无粘连,局部皮肤有无红肿、瘢痕、瘘管等。触诊头颈部淋巴结时,头稍前屈偏向检查一侧,使检查侧局部组织松弛。

触诊腋窝淋巴结时,检查者左手扶着被检查者左前臂,屈肘外展抬高约45°,右手指并拢,掌面贴近胸壁向上直达腋窝顶部,手臂放下靠拢身体,由浅入深滑动触诊。然后依次触诊腋窝后壁、内侧壁、前壁,触诊腋窝前壁时,注意拇指和四指的配合。再翻掌向外,触诊腋窝外侧壁。同法检查右腋窝淋巴结。

触诊左滑车上淋巴结时,用左手扶托被检查者左前臂,并屈肘约90°,以右手小指固定在被检查者的肱骨内上髁,示指、中指及环指并拢,在其上3~4cm处的肱二头肌与肱三头肌的肌沟中,纵行、横行滑动触摸滑车上淋巴结。同法检查右滑车上淋巴结。

触诊腹股沟淋巴结群,应注意腹股沟韧带下方水平组和大隐静脉处垂直组淋巴结群。

观察头发、头颅外形。用双手拨开头发,检查整个头颅有无压痛、包块、损伤等。

检查面神经,视皱额、鼻唇沟、眼裂、闭眼、露齿、鼓腮、吹哨动作左右两侧是否对称。

检查三叉神经,用棉签检查两侧面部对称部位的触觉,并嘱被检查者做咀嚼动作,视动作左右是否对称。

检查视神经,可用近视力表置于33 cm处,遮盖未检查眼,分别检查左右眼在表中能看清的视力。

观察眉毛分布有无脱落,眼睑有无下垂、水肿。嘱被检查者眼睛下视,用右手示指和拇指捏住左上眼睑中部的边缘,轻轻向前牵拉,然后示指向下压,并与拇指配合将睑缘向上捻转,翻转上眼睑。观察上眼睑结膜和穹隆部结膜,提起上眼睑皮肤,使眼睑翻转复原。按同样方法检查右上眼睑。用双手拇指置于下眼睑中部,请受检者向上看,同时向下牵拉睑边缘,观察下眼睑结膜、穹隆部结膜、球结膜及巩膜。请被检查者将眼向外上看,检查者用一手拇指轻压眼内眦下方,即骨性眶缘下内侧挤压泪囊,观察有无分泌物或泪液自上、下泪点溢出。

观察眼球的外形有否凸出或下陷,双侧瞳孔是否等大、等圆。取手电筒,聚光圈后检查对光反射。先查左眼瞳孔,手电光由外向内移动,直接照射瞳孔,并观察左眼瞳孔是否缩小。移开光源后,用手隔开双眼,再次用手电光直接照射左眼瞳孔,并观察右眼瞳孔是否缩小。用同样的方法检查右眼瞳孔。

检查动眼、滑车、外展神经,检查者伸右臂,竖示指,距受检查左眼前约 30~40 cm 处。嘱被检查者双眼注视示指的移动,并告之勿转动头部。示指按水平向左→左上→左下→水平向右→右上→右下,共 6 个方向进行。检查每个方向均代表双眼的一对配偶肌的功能,观察有无眼球运动障碍。

嘱被检查者注视 1 m 以外的示指,然后将示指逐渐地向鼻梁方向移动至距眼球约 5~10 cm 处,观察两眼瞳孔缩小、两侧眼球内聚的变化,称为集合反射。

检查角膜反射时,嘱被检查者向对侧上方注视,用消毒棉签毛由眼角外向内,轻触被检查者的角膜边缘,同时观察两侧眼睑闭合反应。先查左侧,后查右侧。

检查耳廓有无畸形、结节或触痛,请被检查者头部转向右侧,将右手拇指放在耳屏前向前推压,右手示指和中指将耳廓向后上方牵拉,另一手持手电筒,借手电光观察外耳道的皮肤有无溢液。检查乳突有无压痛。先左后右。

观察鼻部皮肤和外形。左手拇指将鼻尖上推,借助手电光观察鼻前庭、鼻中隔和鼻腔有无分泌物。检查者用手指压闭一侧鼻翼,请受检查者呼吸,以判断通气状态。同样方法检查另一侧。检查嗅神经,患者闭目,检查者用手按压病人一侧鼻孔,用盛有气味而无刺激性溶液小瓶(如薄荷水、醋、香水等)置于另一侧鼻孔前,嘱其说出嗅到的气味。同法检查另一侧鼻孔的嗅觉。

检查额窦、筛窦和上颌窦有无压痛。用双手固定于被检查者的两颞侧,将双拇指置于眶上缘内侧的同时向后向上按压,询问有无额窦压痛,两侧有无差别。将手下移,双拇指置于被检查者鼻根部与眼内眦之间,向后内方按压,询问有无筛窦压痛,两侧有无差别。再将两手下移,双拇指置于颧部,同时向后按压,询问有无上颌窦疼痛,两侧有无差别。

检查位听神经,听力可用粗略方法,在静室中被检查者闭目用手指堵塞一侧耳道,检查者用手表或拇指与示指互相摩擦的声音,自1m外逐渐移近耳道,比较两耳测试结果。前庭功能检查观察眼球有无左右、上下、旋转方向的震颤。

观察口唇色泽,有无疱疹、口角糜烂等。取手电筒和消毒压舌板,观察口腔黏膜、牙齿、牙龈,轻轻压迫牙龈,注意有无出血和溢脓。检查上颌第二磨牙对面的颊黏膜上腮腺导管开口处有无分泌物。嘱被检查者张大口并发"a"音,检查者手持压舌板在舌体的前2/3与后1/3交界处迅速下压,借助手电光观察软腭、软腭弓、腭垂、扁桃体和咽后壁。注意有无黏膜充血、红肿、滤泡增生。如果扁桃体增大,则须分度。检查舌下神经请被检查者伸舌,观察伸舌运动有无偏斜的同时观察舌体和舌苔。检查位于耳屏、下颌角、颧弓形成三角区内的腮腺有无肿大。检查舌咽、迷走神经,听发音有无嘶哑,吞咽有无困难,张口发"a"音时,腭垂有无偏斜。

解开衣领,充分暴露颈部。观察颈部皮肤,取上半身与水平面呈45°的半卧位,有无颈静脉充盈、搏动和颈动脉搏动,先左后右。观察甲状腺是否凸出、是否对称。

前面双手触诊法检查甲状腺。检查者右手拇指从胸骨上切迹向上触摸甲状腺峡部在气管前有无增厚,请受检查者做吞咽动作,判断甲状腺峡部有无肿大或肿块。然后用左手拇指施压于一侧甲状软骨,将气管推向对侧,右手示指和中指在左胸锁乳突肌后缘,右手拇指在气管旁,左胸锁乳突肌前缘触诊,使甲状腺左叶在此三指间,以拇指滑动触摸来确定甲状腺的轮廓大小及表面情况,有无肿块、震颤和压痛。请被检查者做吞咽动作,肿大的甲状腺可随吞咽运动上下移位。同法检查甲状腺右叶。位于病人后面触诊甲状腺。被检查者取坐位:检查者用示指从胸骨上切迹向上触摸甲状腺峡部,一手示、中指施压于一侧甲状软骨,将气管推向对侧;另一手拇指在对侧胸锁乳突肌后缘向前推挤甲状腺,示、中指在其前缘气管旁配合吞咽动作触诊甲状腺,用同样方法检查另一侧甲状腺。如有甲状腺肿大,则将听诊器膜型体件放在肿大的甲状腺上,注意有无连续性静脉"嗡鸣音"或收缩期动脉杂音。甲状腺无肿大则无须听诊。

将示指与环指分别放在两侧胸锁关节上,将中指置于气管之前,观察中指与示指、环指间距离,判断有否气管移位。

检查副神经,比较两侧转头、耸肩动作的肌力情况。

(傅志君)

Chapter 3 Head, Neck and Lymph Nodes Exam

Palpate superficial lymph nodes slowly and carefully from the shallow to the deep with the pads of the index, middle and ring fingers. Palpating lymph nodes includes auricular nodes (preauricular nodes, post-auricular nodes, mastoid nodes), the upper and lower group of the deep cervical nodes, submaxillary nodes, submental nodes, supraclavicular nodes (above the patient's collarbone), axillary nodes, epitrochlear lymph nodes, groin lymph nodes, and popliteal lymph nodes. If the lymph nodes are enlarged, please note their location, size, number, hardness, tenderness, mobility, adhesion, fusion, swelling, fistula or scars. For palpating cervical lymph nodes, the examiner may have the patient position his head with his neck slightly flexed forward to keep the skin and muscles relaxed.

The examiner raises the patient's left forearm with his left hand, bending the patient's elbow and rotating his forearm outside to 45 degrees. The examiner places his right palm tightly against the patient's chest wall and then gently moves the palm upwards to the very top of the axilla with all the fingers of his right hand together in order to palpate the axillary nodes. Palpate chains of lymph nodes on the left: posterior, medial, anterior. Be sure that the thumb and the other four fingers cooperate perfectly while palpating the anterior group. Turn the palm outside to feel the lateral group. Use the same method to inspect the patient's right axillary lymph nodes.

The examiner holds the patient's left forearm with his left hand and has the patient bend his elbow to 90 degrees and then fixes his little finger of the right hand on the medial epicondyle of the humerus. The examiner puts index finger, middle finger and ring finger together and feels supratrochlear lymph nodes breadthwise in the groove formed between the biceps and triceps muscles 3 to 4 cm above the medial epicondyle of the humerus. Use the same method to inspect the patient's right supratrochlear lymph nodes.

While palpating groin lymph nodes, the examiner should pay attention to the transverse group which is located below the inguinal ligament and the longitudinal group which runs along the saphenous vein.

Part the hair using both hands to observe the scalp, noting tenderness, lumps or other lesions.

Ask the patient to wrinkle his forehead, close his eyes, show teeth, blow the checks out and purse lips. Note if there is any facial droop or asymmetry.

Cranial nerve V should be briefly checked bilaterally with a fine wisp of cotton, to test the sense of light touch. Ask the patient to perform chewing action. Look for asymmetry.

Use the near eye chart the position of which is calibrated for a distance of 33 cm to test right or left eye respectively. Move the near eye chart far or near until the patient can read it.

Inspect the distribution of eyebrow, the dropping or swelling of eyelids. Instruct the patient to look down, and raise the middle of the left upper eyelid slightly by the index finger and thumb of your right hand as you depress the upper eyelid with your index finger to cooperate with your thumb in order to expose the upper palpebral. Inspect the upper palpebral conjunctivae and the fornical conjunctivae. Inspect the right upper eyelid in the same way.

Instruct the patient to look upward, and put both of your thumbs in the middle of the lower eyelid so that the eyelashes protrude, exposing lower palpebral, fornical, bulbar conjunctiva and sclera. Instruct the patient to look up and outside, and press on the medial canthus slightly with your thumb, that is, you are compressing the lacrimal sac. Look for fluid regurgitation out of the puncta into the eye.

Inspect the shape of the eyes and the size of both pupils. Shine a penlight or the light of the ophthalmoscope into each pupil in turn. Move the penlight from the outer side to the left pupil, and inspect for papillary constriction. Partition the two eyes with one of your hands, and shine the light into the left pupil. Inspect for the right papillary constriction. Use the same method to check the other pupil.

The examiner positions himself in front of the patient and request that, without moving the patient's head, the patient's eyes follow examiner's index finger in six directions. Finger should be 30 ~ 40 cm away from patient's head. The usual format is from mid left, to upper left, lower left, right, upper right and then lower right. Movement of each direction reflects the function of a pair of muscles to inspect for malfunction of eye movement.

The examiner positions himself in front of the patient, asks the patient to look into the distance and then at his finger. The examiner's finger starts from 1 meter away, and then examiner immediately move his finger towards the patient's nose to 5~10 cm away from the patient's eyes. The examiner is observing the patient's eyes for papillary constriction and coordinated movement of both eyes toward fixation at the same near point as the patient focuses on the near subject, which is called accommodation.

Instruct the patient to look opposite upward, and the cornea is touched with a sterilized cotton wisp. An eyelid closure reflex follows almost immediately. Both eyes should be checked, first left and then right.

Inspect the auricle for malformation, tubercle and tenderness. Instruct the patient turn his head to right. Gently pulls the auricle upward, backward with the examiner's right index finger and middle finger. The examiner can observe the skin of the canal with the help of a flashlight. Inspect for tenderness of mastoid. First left and then right.

A view of the nasal cavities is obtained by elevating the tip of the nose by using a thumb and lighting it with a flashlight. Inspect the nasal vestibule, nasal septum and check of secretions in the nasal cavity if present. Test patency by letting the patient inhale through each nostril separately while the other nostril is occluded.

Instruct the patient to close his eyes. The

examiner should block one of the patient's nostrils. Put a bottle of liquid with smell in front of the open nostril and ask the patient to sense the smell. The other nostril should be checked respectively.

The frontal sinuses are palpated at the inner part of the upper border of the bony orbit using the thumb. The pressure is directed upward towards the floor of the sinus. The examiner should ask the patient if there is any tenderness and difference between the left and the right frontal sinuses.

The examiner should move his hands down and press back inward with both thumbs between the middle of nose root and the medial canthus. The examiner should ask the patient if there is any tenderness and difference between the left and the right ethmoid sinus. Simultaneous finger pressure over both maxillae will demonstrate differences in tenderness.

Auditory acuity is tested in each ear separately in a silent room. The examiner should ask the patient to close his eyes and occlude one eye with his fingers while he checks the auditory acuity in the opposite ear. He will ask the patient to respond when the patient hears the sound of the examiner's fingers rubbing together. The examiner should move his fingers from a distance of about 1 meter from the unobstructed ear towards the ear until the patient can distinguish the sound made. The same procedure should be repeated on the opposite ear.

Color, spots, ulceration and any abnormality of the lips should be inspected. Observe the buccal mucosa, teeth, gums using a flashlight and a sterile spatula. Press slightly on the gums and inspect for bleeding and purulence if present. The duct of the parotid gland opens onto the buccal mucosa opposite the upper second molar, inspect for purulence secretion. Instruct the patient to open his mouth and say "a" and then rapidly press the spatula firmly upon the junction of anterior 2/3 and posterior 1/3 of the tongue for inspecting the tonsils, anterior and posterior tonsillar pillars, uvula and posterior pharynx. Inspect for congestion, swelling and spots. If tonsil is enlarged, classify the degree of enlargement. Observe midline protrusion of the tongue (CN XII test). The examiner should ask the patient to stick out his tongue and observe it, tongue fur and midline protrusion. The swelling of the parotid can be observed in the triangle formed by tragus, angle of mandible and zygomatic arch.

Inspect cranial nerve IX, X and inspect for hoarse voice and dysphagia if present. Ask the patient to open his mouth and say "a". Inspect the midline protrusion of uvula.

Have the patient untie his clothes and completely expose his neck. Observe the appearance of the skin of the neck. Have the patient at semireclining position with a 45° between the upper body and level, note the engorgement and pulsation of jugular vein and the pulsation of carotid artery. Inspect the thyroid for enlargement.

Palpate the thyroid from front:

Palpate thyroid isthmus to see if it is thicker by applying pressure with the right thumb upon the thyroid cartilage. Instruct the patient to swallow saliva and inspect for swelling and lumps of thyroid. Later press the thyroid cartilage with your left thumb, and then push the trachea to the opposite side, dislodged lobe of the thyroid can now be palpated between thumb, index and middle finger. Move the thumb to feel the shape and surface of the thyroid. Inspect for the shape and surface of the thyroid. Inspect for lumps, thrills and tenderness. Instruct the patient to swallow and observe the movement of thyroid. Repeat the same method to check the other side.

Palpate the thyroid from behind:

Tell the patient to sit down in the chair. Palpate the thyroid cartilage using the index and the middle finger while the thumb is placed behind the sternomastoid muscle. Tell the patient to swallow as you palpate the gland. Use the same method to check the other side. Apply the diaphragm of the stethoscope over each lobe of the thyroid gland and auscultate for a bruit.

Put the index and ring fingers at the sternoclavicular joints. Palpate trachea or the gaps between the trachea and the joints. Use the middle finger for determining the position/location of the trachea.

Instruct the patient to shrug his shoulder against the resistance, this is to evaluate the strength of trapezius muscle. Now tell him to turn his head to the opposite side against resistance, this is to evaluate the strength of sternocleidomastoid muscle.

Ye Zhibin(叶志斌) Yan Zhenwen(严震文)

第四章 胸廓、肺部检查

被检查者取仰卧位，解开衣服，充分暴露前胸部。视诊皮肤，观察呼吸运动是否均衡、节律是否规整、两侧是否对称，以及肋间隙宽度、胸壁静脉有无曲张。比较胸廓的前后径与左右径，注意胸廓外形的异常改变，如桶状胸、漏斗胸、鸡胸或局部隆起，视诊两侧乳房对称性和乳房皮肤有无异常，乳头的位置、大小和对称性，男性有无乳房增生。

用手掌前部分别触压左右胸廓上、中、下三个部位，注意有无皮下气肿和胸壁触痛。双手按压胸廓两侧，检查胸廓的弹性。用拇指按压胸骨柄及胸骨体的中、下部，询问被检查者有无压痛。女性则常规触诊乳房，取平卧位，肩下垫小枕，使胸部抬起，先查健侧，后查患侧。左乳房检查按外上、尾部、外下、内下、内上顺时针方向由浅入深施加压力滑动触诊，一般以能触及肋骨而不引起疼痛为度，注意乳房有无红、肿、热、痛和包块。触诊乳晕和乳头，则用拇指和示指同时轻压乳头两侧对应部位，注意有无硬结和分泌物。右乳房检查按外上、尾部、外下、内下、内上顺序，循逆时针方向进行触诊。

检查胸廓扩张度，当触诊前胸时，两手掌及伸展的手指置于胸廓前下外侧的对称位置，左右拇指指尖分别沿两侧肋缘指向剑突，拇指间距约

2 cm,然后嘱被检查者做深呼吸动作,比较两手的动度是否一致。触诊背部时,双手平置于第 10 肋骨水平,双拇指平行地放于受检者后正中线两侧数厘米处,嘱受检者深呼吸,观察拇指间随胸廓扩张而与后正中线分离的距离是否一致。

将双手掌置于被检查者胸部的对称位置,嘱其以同等强度发"yi"长音,并将双手手掌作一次交换,以排除两手感觉的误差。检查前后胸部上、中、下各部位,比较两侧相应部位语音震颤的异同,注意有无增强、减弱。背部肩胛间区用手掌尺侧缘进行触诊。

双手掌置于被检查者左右胸廓前下侧部,嘱其深呼吸,触诊有无胸膜摩擦感。

检查前胸时双臂平放在身体两侧,检查胸部叩诊音分布,以胸骨角为标志,确定肋间隙。左手中指为板指与肋骨平行,用右手中指指端叩击板指第二指骨前端,每次叩 2~3 次,叩击后右手中指应立即抬起,以免影响叩诊音的判断。由第 1 肋间至第 4 肋间,按由外向内、自上而下、两侧对照的原则叩诊。在叩肩胛间区时,被检查者双手抱肘,板指可与脊柱并行。注意叩诊音改变及板指的震动感。

肺上界叩诊,被检查者取坐位,检查者立于被检查者身后,用间接叩诊法自斜方肌前缘中央部开始向外叩诊,由清音变浊音是肺上界外侧终点,然后转向内侧叩诊,由清音变为浊音是肺上界内侧终点。此清音带宽度为肺尖宽度,又称 Kronig 峡,正常约为 5 cm。

肺下界叩诊,在双侧锁骨中线、腋中线、肩胛线上叩诊。被检查者平静呼吸,检查者板指贴于肋间隙,自上而下,由清音叩到浊音时翻转板指,取板指中部用标记笔作标记,数肋间隙并作记录。正常人平静呼吸在锁骨中线、腋中线和肩胛线上肺下界分别是第6、第8和第10肋间隙。

肺下界移动范围叩诊,沿左肩胛线自上而下,叩出平静呼吸时的肺下界。嘱被检查者作深吸气后屏住呼吸,迅速沿左肩胛线向下叩诊由清音变为浊音时,翻转板指,在其中点用标记笔作一标记。恢复平静呼吸,再嘱其深呼气后屏气,迅速沿左肩胛线自下而上叩诊,当浊音变为清音时,翻转板指,再作标记,嘱被检查者恢复正常呼吸。用直尺测量两个标记间的距离,即左侧肺下界移动范围。同法再叩及右肺下界移动范围,测量后并作记录。正常人肺下界移动范围 6~8cm。

肺部听诊用听诊器膜型体件在前胸按肺尖,左、右锁骨中线上、中、下部,侧胸按左、右腋中线上、下部,背部按左、右肩胛间区上、下,左、右肩胛线上、下至少20个听诊点。比较两侧呼吸音有无异常变化,是否有呼吸音以外的附加音(干、湿啰音)。嘱被检查者作深吸气动作。于左、右前下侧胸部听诊有无胸膜摩擦音。

于前、后胸部上、中、下各触诊部位嘱被检查者以同等强度发"yi"长音,听诊两侧语音共振的变化。

(傅志君)

Chapter 4 Examination of Thorax and Lung

Ask the patient to lie in the supine position, tell him to take off the clothes and expose prothorax thoroughly. Carefully inspect whether the respiratory movement is stable, regular and symmetrical. Inspect varicose veins on chest wall if any. Examine the width of intercostal space. Compare the anteroposterior diameter with transverse diameter of chest wall, inspect whether the form of chest wall have any abnormalities, such as barrel chest, funnel chest, pigeon chest and local eminence. Inspect if both the breasts are symmetric or not, examine the skin, examine the location, size and symmetry of the nipples, check for mammoplasia in males if present.

Palpate the superior, middle and inferior parts of both sides of chest wall using anterior part of your palms. Check for subcutaneous emphysema or tenderness. Palpate the bilateralism of chest wall with both hands to check the elasticity of the chest wall. Ask the patient whether there is tenderness while palpating the manubrium of sternum, the middle and inferior parts of the body of sternum with the thumb.

As for female, breasts should be palpated routinely. Ask the patient to lie in the supine position. Put a small pillow under her shoulder to elevate the thoracic parts. If noticeable examine the healthy side first, then the ill side. Check the upper outer quadrant, tail, lower outer quadrant, lower inner quadrant and upper inner quadrant of left breast one by one clockwise from superficial to deep. Softly palpate till you can touch the ribs but this should be gentle enough not to cause pain. Inspect whether there is flare, engorgement, cauma, pain or mass on the breasts. While palpating the areolas of breast and nipples, press the corresponding parts of nipples slightly with thumb and forefinger together to see whether there is induration or secretion. Palpate the upper outer quadrant, tail, lower outer quadrant, lower inner quadrant and upper inner quadrant of right breast in anticlockwise direction.

Inspect the expandability of thoracic cage. While palpating prothorax, both palms and stretched fingers should be put on the lower lateral parts of prothorax symmetrically and two thumbtips should be directed towards xiphoid process following both costal margins respectively, the distance of two thumbs should be about two centimeters. Then ask the patient to breathe deeply, meanwhile compare whether the motions of both hands are consistent. When palpating the back, put both hands gently on the patient's rib cage at the 10th costal level from behind with fingers between the ribs, thumbs on the places few centimeters away from the posterior median line and parallel to the spinal column, and have patient breathe in and out. Observe whether the distance between the thumbs and the posterior median line are consistent while thoracic cage expanding.

Put the palms on the symmetric places of the patient's chest wall. Ask the patient to pronounce prolonged "yi" with the same loudness. Then interchange the two palms to exclude the error of the sensation. Check the superior, middle and inferior parts of prothorax and metathorax to compare whether the vocal fremitus on corresponding places of both sides are different, check whether they are enhanced or weakened. Palpate the interscapular region on back with ulnar side of palms.

Put the palms on the patient's anteroinferior parts of the thoracic cage respectively, then ask the patient to breathe in deeply, palpate whether there is sense of pleural friction.

Ask the patient to put both arms at the side while you are checking the prothorax. Examine the distribution of percussion sounds on thorax, and define the intercostal space according to the angle of sternum. Place the middle finger of the left hand on the intercostal space parallel with ribs. Percuss the anterior part of the second phalange of sensing finger with the midfingertip of the right hand. Each point should be percussed two or three times. After the percussion, you should raise the middle finger of the right hand immediately to avoid affecting the judgement of the percussion sound. You should percuss from the first intercostal space to the fourth comparatively and symmetrically from top to bottom and from lateral to medial. Ask the patient to take the position of cubital fixing ring. When percussing interscapular area, middle finger should be parallel to spine. Pay attention to the sound and the feeling of sensing finger.

When percussing the upper boundary of the lung, let the patient take the sitting position. The examiner should stand behind the patient, percuss from the middle part of the anterior border of the trapezius muscle to the outside by mediate percussion. When resonant note changes to dullness, it shows that you have reached the end point of the lateral upper boundary of the lungs. From there you should percuss to inside until resonant note changes to dullness, it represents that you have reached the end point of the wall upper boundary of the lung.

The width of the resonant note is the width of the apex of lung which is also named Kronig isthmus and the normal range of it is about five centimeters.

When percussing the bottom of lung, you should percuss on midclavicular, midaxillary and scapular lines of both sides. Ask the patient to respire smoothly, the sensing finger of the examiner should stick to intercostal space, then percuss from top to bottom. Don't remove the finger until resonant note changes to dullness. Mark the point with a marker pen, then count and record the number of the intercostal spaces. Normally the lower borders of lungs on midclavicular, midaxillary and scapular line are on the level of fifth, seventh and tenth intercostal space respectively when respiring smoothly.

To measure the degree of excursion of lower border of left lung, you should percuss from top to bottom direction following the left scapular line to percuss for base of the lungs during normal breathing at first. Then ask the patient to take a deep breath and hold it. Percuss following the left scapular line downward quickly. When resonant note changes to dullness, remove the finger and mark the changing point with a marker. Ask the patient to breathe smoothly, and then ask the patient to exhale completely and hold it. Percuss following the left scapular line upward quickly. When dull sound changes to resonant note, mark the point again. Ask the patient to breathe smoothly. Note the difference between the two points, which should be 6~8 cm. Measure the degree of excursion of lower border of right lung in the same way.

Auscultate the lung by using the diaphragm of the stethoscope, from apex of lung, then the superior, middle and inferior part of left and right midclavicular line on the prothorax, superior, inferior part of left and right midaxillary line on lateralthorax, superior and inferior part of left and right interscapular region, superior and inferior part of left and right scapular line on back, which amount to no less than twenty auscultation points. Compare whether respiratory sounds on both sides are normal, whether there are adventitious sounds besides respiratory sounds (such as rhonchi and moist rales). Instruct the patient to inspire deeply and auscultate whether there is pleuritic rub on anteroinferior parts of both sides of the chest.

Ask the patient to pronounce prolonged "yi" with the same loudness when the examiner auscultates superior, middle and inferior parts of prothorax and metathorax. Compare resonance of both sides bilaterally and symmetrically.

Wang Baoqing (王葆青)

第五章　心脏、血管检查

被检查者取仰卧位。检查者下蹲,以切线方向观察心前区是否隆起,观察心尖搏动的位置、强弱和范围,以及心前区有无异常搏动。

先用右手掌置于心前区,然后用手掌尺侧小鱼际触诊,注意心尖搏动的位置和有无震颤,最后用并拢的示指和中指的指腹确定心尖搏动的位置、范围、强弱,有无抬举性搏动,确定心前区有无异常搏动(包括剑突下搏动)。用手掌在心底部和胸骨左缘第4肋间触诊,注意有无震颤及心包摩擦感。心包摩擦感于前倾坐位收缩期呼气末更明显。必要时用手掌尺侧(小鱼际)确定震颤的具体位置,判定收缩期还是舒张期。

心脏叩诊先叩左界,从心尖搏动最强点外侧2~3 cm处开始,沿肋间由外向内,采用轻叩法,叩诊音由清音变为浊音时,翻转板指,在板指中点用标记笔作标记。如此自下而上,叩至第2肋间。叩右界则先沿右锁骨中线,自上而下,叩诊音由清音变浊音时,即为肝上界,于其上一肋间(一般为第4肋间)由外向内叩出浊音界,自下而上,逐个肋间叩诊,于第2、3肋间由外向内叩出浊音界(此为相对浊音界),并分别作标记。然后标出前正中线和左锁骨中线,用直尺测量左、右心浊音界各标记点距前正中线的垂直距离和左锁骨中线与前正中线间的距离。

心脏听诊先将听诊器膜型体件置心尖搏动最强的部位,听诊1分钟,注意心率、心律、心音强度和心音分裂、额外心音、杂音、心包摩擦音,然后依次在肺动脉瓣区(胸骨左缘第2肋间)、主动脉瓣区(胸骨右缘第2肋间)、主动脉瓣第二听诊区(胸骨左缘第3肋间)、三尖瓣区(胸骨下端左缘,即胸骨左缘第4、5肋间)听诊。注意A_2与P_2的强度比较,心音分裂与呼吸的关系,如听到杂音,应认真辨别其最响的部位、时期、性质、传导、强度及与体位、呼吸、运动的关系。在胸骨左缘第3、4肋间听诊心包摩擦音,听诊左、右颈部大血管有无杂音。

比较双侧桡动脉搏动是否一致,有无交替脉。请被检查者深吸气,检查有无奇脉。左手示指、中指、环指指腹触于桡动脉处,紧握被检查者右手腕,将被检查者前臂高举过头,感觉桡动脉的搏动,判断有无水冲脉。用手指轻压被检查者指甲末端,观察甲床有无红白交替现象,即毛细血管搏动征。

比较两侧股动脉的搏动是否存在,搏动强度是否一致,并将听诊器膜型体件置于股动脉搏动处,听诊有无射枪音,稍加压力,注意有无 Duroziez 双重杂音。

双手同时触摸两侧第1、2趾骨间足背动脉,并作比较,搏动是否正常。

(傅志君)

Chapter 5　Cardiovascular Examination

Instruct the patient to lie in the supine position. The examiner inspects the precordium at a tangent to identify whether the precordium is hunched, the location, intensity and range of apical impulse, and whether there is an abnormal impulse.

First, the palm of the right hand is placed at the area of precordium, then use the hypothenar to palpate apical impluse and detect if there is any thrill present. After that, try to pin down the precise location, range and intensity of the apical impulse with the tip of the index and middle fingers, especially the palpable heave and the pathologic impulses (including the impulse under the xiphoid). Palpate the second left intercostal space, the second right intercostal space and the forth left intercostal space to feel for the thrill and the pericardial friction. The pericardial friction is felt more easily when the patient is sitting and leaning forward in late expiration and systole. If necessary, it is recommended to identify the exact location of the thrill and whether it happens in diastole or systole.

Generally, percussion of the heart starts on the left side of the chest, 2 ~ 3 cm outside the point of maximum impulse, tap along the intercostals towards to the left sternal edge, and stop when the quality of the sound changes from the resonant sound to the dull one and mark this point. Tap continuously as it progresses upwards to the second intercostal space. Then percuss the right border: tap continuously along the right mid-clavicula line downwards. It is the upper border of the liver where the sound changes. Move one intercostal upward (usually the forth intercostal space) and tap along the intercostals from the outside to the inside to delineate the right border of the heart just as it is done to delineate the left border of the heart. Mark the anterior midline and the left mid clavicula line. Then measure the plumb distance between the left border and the anterior midline, the plumb distance between the right border and the anterior midline and the plumb distance between the anterior midline and the left mid clavicula line.

Auscultate with diaphragm of the stethoscope. Engage the diaphragm of the stethoscope and place it firmly over the point of maximum impulse over one minute to identify the rate, rhythm, loudness of the heart sound, the split of the heart sound, extra heart sounds, murmurs and the pericardial friction rubs. Then move it orderly to the pulmonic area (the second left intercostal space), the aortic area (the second right intercostal space), the second aortic area (the third left intercostal space) and the tricuspid area (the forth or fifth left intercostal space). Compare the loudness of A_2 (aortic valve closure) and P_2 (pulmonic valve closure) and pay attention to the relationship between the split of the heart sound and the respiration. When murmurs are detected, close attention should be given to the location, timing, quality, radiation, loudness of the murmurs and the relationship between murmurs and the positions of the body, the respiration and movements. The pericardial friction rubs are usually detected at the third or forth left intercostal space. Auscultation over the carotid arteries to find if there is carotid bruits.

Compare the intensity of radial artery impulses of both sides to find if they are symmetric and if there are pulsus alternans. In deep inspiration, paradoxical pulses can be detected. Palpate the radial artery impulses with the left index, middle and ring fingers circling the right wrist of the patient and elevating the arm above the head to find if there are water-hammer pulses. Press the nail bed of any finger slightly to see if there are capillary pulsations (the "red-white commutation" phenomenon).

Compare the intensity of femoral artery impulses of both sides to find if they are symmetric and place the diaphragm of the stethoscope over the impulses to find if there are pistol shot sounds and the Duroziez sign with a heavier application of the stethoscope.

Compare the intensity of both dorsum pedes artery impulses between the great and the second toe to find if the intensity is normal and if they are symmetric.

Zhu Wenqing(朱文青)

第六章 腹部检查

嘱被检查者取仰卧位,充分暴露腹部。检查者蹲下平视腹部外形是否平坦。视诊腹部皮肤、腹式呼吸运动是否存在或有无腹部外形异常,有无腹壁静脉曲张、胃肠型或蠕动波,脐部有无凸出等。

请被检查者屈膝并稍分开,使腹肌松弛。用全手掌放于腹壁上,感觉腹肌紧张度,并使患者适应片刻。然后轻柔地进行腹部浅触诊,腹部压陷约 1~2 cm。先触诊未诉病痛的部位,一般自左下腹开始滑行触诊,然后沿逆时针方向移动,同时观察被检查者的反应及面部表情。检查者右手前臂与腹部表面呈同一水平,先用全手掌放于腹壁上,使被检查者适应片刻,以掌指关节和腕关节协调动作自左下腹逆时针方向进行触诊,检查每个区域后,检查者手应提起并离开腹壁,不能停留在腹壁上移动。注意腹壁的紧张度、抵抗感、表浅的压痛、包块、搏动和腹壁上的肿物。用指尖深压位于脐与右髂前上棘连线中、外 1/3 交界处的 McBurney 点,当检查腹部出现压痛后,触诊手在腹壁上停留片刻后突然将手抬起,以检查有无反跳痛。再作深触诊,腹壁压陷约 2 cm 以上,可单手、左手与右手重叠,以并拢的手指末端逐渐加压触摸深部脏器,同浅触诊一样,一般自左下腹开始,按逆时针方向进行。如果触及肿物或包块,须注意其位置、大小、形态、质地、压痛、搏动、移动度及与腹壁的关系。

双手触诊法检查肝脏。嘱被检查者张口作较深的腹式呼吸,检查者用左手拇指置于季肋部,其余四指置于右腰背部,以限制右下胸扩张,增加膈下移的幅度。右手四指并拢,掌指关节伸直,与肋缘大致平行地放在右上腹部(或脐右侧)估计肝下缘的下方,在被检查者呼气时手指沿右锁骨中线压向腹部深处,吸气时手指向上迎触下移的肝缘。如此反复进行,手指逐渐向肋缘移动直至触及肝缘或肋缘为止。注意吸气时手指上抬的速度要落后于腹壁的抬起。如果肋下触及肝脏,宜在右锁骨中线叩出肝上界并测量肝脏的上下径间距离,以排除肝脏下移。然后在前正中线上触诊肝脏,一般从脐部开始,自下向上滑行移动,与呼吸运动配合,测量肝缘与剑突或剑突根部间的距离。触及肝脏除测量肝脏的大小外,还应注意其质地、表面、边缘、压痛、搏动感、摩擦感及肝震颤等。肝脏肿大者作肝颈静脉回流征检查,即用手掌压迫右上腹部肿大的肝脏,观察颈静脉,如出现颈静脉怒张更加明显,则为肝颈静脉回流征阳性。正常人肝脏在右锁骨中线肋缘下<1 cm,剑突下<3 cm,质软、表面光滑、无压痛。

脾脏双手触诊法,左手掌置于被检查者左腰部第9～11肋处,试从后向前托起脾脏,右手掌平放于腹壁上,与肋弓大致呈垂直方向。一般从髂前上棘水平(或估计脾下缘的下方)开始,两手配合,随呼吸运动深部滑行向肋弓方向触诊脾脏,直至触及脾缘或左肋缘。触诊不满意时,可嘱被检查者取右侧卧位,右下肢伸直,左下肢屈曲使腹部皮肤松弛,再作触诊。如脾脏肿大,则测量甲乙线、甲丙线和丁戊线;除大小外,还应注意脾脏的质地、表面情况、有无压痛及摩擦感等。正常人脾脏常不能触及。

被检查者仍取仰卧位,两腿屈起稍分开。于右肋缘下腹直肌外缘单手滑行触诊有无胆囊肿大,如触及囊性显著肿大胆囊,但无压痛称为Courvoisier征。正常人胆囊不能触及。Murphy征检查,以左手掌平放于被检查者右季肋区下部,以拇指指腹勾压腹直肌外缘与肋弓交界处,其余四指与肋骨交叉。然后嘱其做深吸气,同时注意被检查者的面部表情,询问有无疼痛。因疼痛而突然中止吸气动作,为 Murphy 征阳性。肾脏触诊可取卧位双腿屈曲并做较深呼吸,检查者以左手掌向上托住被检查者右腰部,右手掌平放于右上腹部,手指方向大致平行于右肋缘而稍横向。于被检查者吸气时双手夹触肾脏。触诊左肾时,左手越过患者前方而托住左腰部,右手掌横置于患者左上腹部,依前法双手触诊左肾。正常人肾脏一般不易触及,有时可触及右肾下极。如在深吸气时能触到 1/2 以上肾脏即为肾下垂。如肾下垂明显并能在腹腔各个方向移动时称为游走肾。

双手拇指依次深压两侧肋弓第 10 肋骨下缘偏内（即前肾点）、脐水平腹直肌外缘（上输尿管点）和髂前上棘水平腹直肌外缘（中输尿管点），注意有无压痛。检查肝区叩击痛，用左手掌平放在右季肋区，右手握拳由轻到中等力量叩击左手背，询问叩击时有无疼痛。

液波震颤检查时，检查者左手掌轻贴被检查者右侧腹壁，右手四指并拢屈曲，用右手指指腹叩击左侧腹壁。如左手掌有波动感，为排除腹壁本身振动的传导，则请被检查者或助手用右手掌尺侧缘压在脐部腹正中线上，再叩击对侧腹壁，当腹水 >3 000 ml 时贴于右腹壁的手掌仍有被液体冲击的感觉，则为液波震颤阳性。

检查者左耳凑近被检查者上腹部，右手示、中、环三指并拢置于上腹部，手指与腹壁呈 70°角作数次急速有力的冲击动作，如闻及气体和液体相互撞击的声音即为振水音。若空腹或餐后 6~8 小时以上，仍有此音，则提示幽门梗阻或胃扩张。

腹部叩诊音的检查同浅触诊，从左下腹开始，以逆时针方向叩诊，发现其有无异常的浊音或实音。腹部的大部分区域为鼓音，肝、脾所在部位为浊音。

肝上界叩诊，用间接叩诊法，肝上界在右锁骨中线、右腋中线、右肩胛线上分别为第 5、7、10 肋间，不同体型、胖瘦者可略有变化，正常人在右锁骨中线肝脏上、下径间距离为9~11 cm。脾脏叩诊常在左腋中线第9~11肋之间用轻叩法，其长度为4~7 cm，前方不超过腋前线。胃泡鼓音区(Traube区)位于左前胸下部肋缘以上，约呈半圆形，大小受胃内含气量多少而定。

移动性浊音的叩诊，先从脐部开始，沿脐水平向左侧方向移动。当叩诊音由鼓音变为浊音时，板指位置固定，嘱被检查者右侧卧位，稍停片刻，重新叩诊该处，听取音调是否变为鼓音。然后向右侧移动叩诊，移动不便时可改变指尖方向，继续叩诊直达浊音区，叩诊板指固定位置，嘱被检查者向左侧翻身180°呈左侧卧位，停留片刻后再次叩诊，听取叩诊音之变化。当游离腹水＞1 000 ml时，可出现浊音区随体位移动而变动之现象，为移动性浊音阳性。

检查肾脏病变时，被检查者采用坐位或侧卧位，用双拇指按压背部第12肋骨与脊柱夹角的顶点(即肋脊点)和第12肋骨与腰肌外缘的夹角顶点(即肋腰点)，同时询问被检查者有无疼痛。用左手掌平放在左肋脊角处，右手握拳用轻到中等的力量叩击左手背，询问有无疼痛，即肾区叩击痛。然后检查右侧肾区有无叩击痛。

右下腹听诊肠鸣音1分钟。正常情况下肠鸣音每分钟4~5次，如每分钟10次以上称肠鸣音活跃。如次数增多且肠鸣音响亮高亢，甚至呈叮当声或金属音，称肠鸣音亢进。在中腹部，左、右上腹部，两下腹部，分别听诊腹主动脉、肾动脉和髂动脉部位的血管杂音。在腹壁静脉曲张患者的上腹部和脐周听诊静脉杂音(Cruveilhier-Baumgarten 综合征)。在妊娠 5 个月的患者可在左、右下腹部听到胎儿心音,在肝区和脾区听诊有无摩擦音。鉴于腹部触诊和叩诊可能影响肠鸣音的活跃程度,可根据专科情况,腹部检查改为视、听、触、叩的顺序进行。

(傅志君)

Chapter 6 Abdominal Examination

Ask the examinee to lie flat on his back with abdomen exposed fully. Examiner should inspect for the scars, striae, hernias, vascular changes, lesions, or rashes, movement associated with peristalsis or pulsations. Note the abdominal contour for flatness, scaphoid, or protuberance.

Ask the examinee to bend both the knees and open a little to relax his abdominal muscles. Examiner should put his hand on the abdominal wall with his right forearm at the same level of the surface of abdomen, to feel the tense of the muscle and let the examinee adapt the stimuli. Now proceed with the light palpation tenderly, pressing the abdominal wall down 1 ~ 2 cm. Firstly, palpitation should avoid the area that the examinee complain of pain. Use the metacarpophalangeal joint and wrist joint to palpate in phase from the left lower quadrant retrorse. Every time after the examination of an area, the examiner should lift his hand off the abdominal wall, avoid moving in the surface and observe the reflection and facial expression of the examinee since the most sensitive indicator of tenderness is the patient's facial expression. Notice for tense, resistance, tenderness, mass, pulsation and mass in the abdominal wall. Use the tips of fingers to pressure deeply the McBurney point lying in the boundary between the middle and external 1/3 of right anterior superior iliac spine line. For checking the rebound tenderness, press deeply on the abdomen with your hand, after a moment, examiner should quickly release pressure and lift the hand immediately to observe whether rebound tenderness present or not. If it hurts more when you release, the patient has rebound tenderness. Now proceed with the deep palpation on the abdomen wall pressured more than 2 cm. You can use one hand or with two hands lapping over, use your fingers to touch the deep organs with the gentle pressure gradually. Start from the left lower quadrant retrorse. If you touch a mass, you should describe the location, size, texture, tenderness, pulsations, mobility and its relation with abdominal wall.

Palpate the liver with both hands. Ask the examinee to open his mouth to take a deep abdominal breath. The examiner should put his left thumb just below the right costal margin and press firmly, and the other four fingers on the back of right waist to limit the movement of lower right lung and to increase the extent of diaphragm downwards. Close the four fingers of right hand, stretch the metacarpophalangeal joint and put on the right upper quadrant (or right to the umbilicus), parallelling with the rib margin, about the lower edge of the liver. The fingers press deeply when the examinee is expiring and up to the edge of liver when inspinning. Repeat until the fingers touch the edge of liver or the rib margin. Be careful that speed of lift fingers should slower than the lift of the wall. If the liver is palpable, it would be better to percuss the upper border of the liver and measure the distance between the upper and lower border to exclude the descending of liver. And then palpate the liver along the anterior median line. Generally start from the umbilicus, slowly move upwards in rhythm with the breath, and measure the distance between the lower border of the liver and xiphoid. Notice the texture, surface, edges, tenderness, pulsations, friction and thrill if any. You should perform the hepatojugular reflux if the liver is enlarged. Put your hand to the enlarged liver in the right upper quadrant and observe the jugular vein. If the vein distend obviously, it means hepatojugular reflux positive. Normal anatomy of liver is nearly 1 cm beyond the rib margin in the midclavicular line and less than 3 cm beyond the xiphoid, soft, lubricous surface and without tenderness.

Palpate the spleen with both hands. Place the left hand on the left waist between 9~11 rib to lift the spleen ahead and place the right palm on the abdominal wall flatly, vertical with the rib arc. Generally, start from the anterosuperior iliac spine level (or estimate the lower of the spleen margin), use both hands to cooperate and make deep slip movement to palpate the spleen with the breath until touch the edge of the spleen or the left rib margin. If the palpation is not satisfactory, you can ask the examinee to lie on the right side, stretch the right lower extremity and bend the left lower extremity to relax the skin of the wall and palpate again. If the spleen is enlarged, measure the AB line, the AC line and the DE line. Notice the size, texture, surface, tenderness and friction if any. A normal spleen is not palpable.

Palpate the gall bladder using a hand at the right rib margin and the external edge of rectus abdominis. It is called Courvoisier sign if you touch the enlarged cystic gall bladder without tenderness. A normal gall bladder is not palpable. Murphy's sign: put the left palm on the lower quadrant of the right rib margin, and use the pad of thumb to draw the boundary between outer edge of rectus abdominis muscle and rib bow, and the other four fingers across the ribs. Ask the examinee to inspire deeply, observe his facial expression and ask whether there is a pain or not. Once the examinee stops inspiration due to pain, the Murphy's sign is positive.

Palpation of kidney: Ask the examinee to lie down, bend his knees and tell him to take deep breath. The examiner puts his left palm to hold the examinee's right waist, and his right palm on the abdominal wall flatly with the fingers paralleling with the right rib margin and a little breadthwise. Bring two hands closer and palpate the kidney when the examinee is inspiring. When palpate the left kidney, the examiner's left palm cross the examinee and hold his waist, put the right palm on the left upper abdominal wall, and use the same method to palpate the left kidney. A normal kidney is not palpable, and sometimes we can palpate the right lower border of kidney. Once you palpate the half of kidney when deep expiration it is called nephroptosia. If the nephroptosia is obvious and can float in every direction in the abdominal cavity it is called floating kidney.

Use your thumbs to press the following points deeply and in order: the inside of lower edge of the 10th rib (the anterior kidney point), outer edge of rectus abdominis muscle at the level of umbilicus (upper ureter point) and outer edge of rectus abdominis muscle at the level of anterosuperior iliac spine (middle ureter point), noticing that whether it pains or not.

Percussion of the liver: the palm of left hand is applied anteriorly to the lower ribs of the right hemithorax. The back of the applied hand is struck lightly with the fist of the right hand and ask the examinee whether it pains or not.

Fluid thrill: the examiner should put his left palm on the right abdominal wall and bends his four fingers of right hand, tap the opposite flank of the abdomen. Once there is the feeling of fluctuating, ask the examinee or the assistant to place the ulnar part of his hand firmly in the midline of the abdomen to exclude the transmission of the thrill from abdominal wall itself. When there is more than 3,000 ml fluid in the abdominal cavity, the palm putting on the right abdominal wall can feel the impact from fluid and it is called fluid thrill positive.

The examiner brings his left ear close to the upper abdomen of the examinee, press the upper abdomen with his index, middle and ring fingers rapidly and strongly in the angle of 70 degrees. Once hear the sound of bounce from gas and fluid it is called succussion splash. Once this kind of sound can be heard while fasting or 6 ~ 8 hours postprandial, it indicates pyloric obstruction or gastric dilatation.

Use the same method to perform the percussion of abdomen with light palpation, starting from the left lower abdomen and percussing anticlockwise to identify the abnormal dullness or flatness. Tympany is the most common percussion sound in the abdomen. Organs will appear as dullness.

Percussion of the top edge of liver: indirect percussion. The top edge of liver lies in the 5th, 7th and 10th rib in the right midclavicular line, right middle axillary line, right scapular line respectively, vary a little according to the shape. The distance between top and lower edge of liver is 9 ~ 11 cm in the right midclavicular line. Use light percussion to measure the spleen between the 9th and 11th rib in the left middle axillary line, the length is about 4 ~ 7 cm and the anterior edge does not exceed beyond the anterior axillary line. Percussion of gastric tympany: Traube semilunar space lies above the left anterior chest and lower rib margin, with semilunar shape and the size is determined by the air volum in the gastric.

Shifting dullness: With the patient lying in supine position, begin percussion at the level of the umbilicus and proceed down laterally. When you reach a point where the sound changes from tympanitic to dull, mark this point and then have the patient roll into a lateral decubitus position (i. e. onto either their right or left sides). Repeat percussion, beginning at the top of the patient's now upturned side and moving down towards the umbilicus. If there is ascites, fluid more than 1,000 ml, the place at which sound changes from tympanitic to dull will therefore have shifted upwards (towards the umbilicus) and it is called shifting dullness positive.

Kidney: Instruct the examinee to sit or lie on his one side, and the examiner presses the angle point made by the 12th rib and spine in the back (costovertebral angle) and the angle point of 12th rib and the outer edge of trunk muscle (costotrunk angle), at the same time ask the examinee whether he/she feels the pain or not. Apply the left palm on the left costovertebral angle and struck the back of left hand with fist of right hand lightly to moderately and ask whether there is a pain or not, this is the kidney percussion pain. And proceed the same way to the right side of kidney.

Auscultate the bowel sound for 1 minute. 4 ~ 5 times movements a minute is normal. It is called bowel sound activity. Once you hear more times and the tone is high and sonorous, it is called increased bowel sound. Auscultate the abdominal aorta, renal artery and iliac artery to identify vessel murmurs in the middle and the bilateral upper and lower abdomen. Auscultate to the vein murmur in the upper abdomen and peri-umbilicus of the abdominal wall varicosity patient (Cruveilhier-Baumgarten syndrome). You can hear the fetal heart sound in the bilateral lower abdomen of 5 months above pregnant patients. Auscultate the area of liver and spleen to identify whether it has friction or not. Since the palpation and percussion may influence the activity of bowel sound, abdominal physical examination should be performed in order of inspection, auscultation, palpation and percussion.

Lai Yanni(赖雁妮)

第七章 脊柱、四肢、神经反射检查

揭开被子,去枕,嘱被检查者下肢自然伸直,颈部放松,检查者左手托住被检查者枕部,右手放在其胸前,左手使被检查者头部前屈做被动屈颈动作,测试颈肌抵抗力,有无颈项强直;再次被动屈颈,观察两膝关节和髋关节的活动,如有屈曲则为 Brudzinski 征阳性。先使被检查者左髋、左膝关节屈曲成直角后,检查者左手置于膝关节上,右手置踝部并抬高小腿。正常人膝关节可伸达 135°以上,如伸膝受限伴有疼痛,而且对侧膝关节屈曲则为 Kernig 征阳性,同样方法查右侧下肢,这些均为脑膜刺激征象。

请被检查者取坐位,前、后、左、右活动颈部及腰部,观察脊柱的活动度,有无活动受限。检查者用手指沿脊柱的棘突以适当的压力从上向下划压,观察划压后皮肤出现的红色充血线,判断脊柱有无侧弯。检查者用拇指自上而下逐个按压脊柱棘突及椎旁肌肉直至骶部,询问有无压痛。先用间接叩击法,嘱被检查者坐正,将左手掌置于被检查者头顶部,右手半握拳以小鱼际部位叩击左手背。观察被检查者有无疼痛,疼痛部位多提示病变位置。然后用叩诊锤直接叩击胸椎和腰椎各椎体的棘突,询问有无叩击痛。如有叩击痛,则以第 7 颈椎棘突为骨性标记,计数病变椎体位置。

请被检查者取仰卧位,取棉签分别沿肋缘下、脐水平、腹股沟上,由外向内轻划刺激腹壁皮肤,先左后右、左右对比,检查上、中、下腹壁反射是否引出,正常反应见局部腹肌收缩。

盖好被子,视诊上肢皮肤、关节、手指及指甲。

请被检查者活动上肢,观察肩、肘、腕、指关节有无畸形,有无肝掌。检查肩关节前屈、后伸、外展、内收、旋转,肘关节屈伸、旋转,腕关节掌屈、背伸、外展、内收,指关节屈曲、伸展的活动功能有无障碍和出现疼痛。检查者右手置被检查者左前臂外侧,并使其左前臂处外旋位,嘱被检查者用力屈肘;检查者右手置被检查者左前臂外侧,嘱其用力做伸肘运动,观察肌肉克服阻力的力量,即肌力,正常肌力为 5 级。相同方法测试右臂肌力,并与左侧作比较。请被检查者双手紧握检查者示指和中指,检查者用力回抽,以比较双侧握力。放松上肢比较两侧肌张力。

检查者以左手托住被检查者半屈曲的肘部,将左拇指置于肱二头肌肌腱上,然后用叩诊锤叩击检查者拇指,观察前臂快速屈曲动作,即肱二头肌反射。用叩诊锤直接叩击尺骨鹰嘴上方的肱三头肌肌腱,观察前臂的伸展动作,为肱三头肌反射。被检查者外展上臂,半屈曲肘部,检查者使被检查者腕部桡侧面向上,并使腕关节自然下垂,用叩诊锤叩击桡骨茎突上方,观察前臂旋前、屈肘动作,为桡骨膜反射。检查者左手握住被检查者腕关节上方,右手以中指及示指夹持被检查者中指,并稍向上提,使腕部处于轻度过伸位,然后以拇指迅速向下弹刮患者中指指甲,如果其余四指有轻微的掌屈动作,则为 Hoffmann 征阳性。同样的方法检查右侧。

暴露下肢,视诊双下肢皮肤、下肢静脉,观察髋、膝、踝、跖关节有无畸形,检查髋关节屈曲、伸展、外展、内收、旋转,膝关节伸屈、旋转,踝、跖关节背屈、跖屈的活动功能有无障碍和出现疼痛。触压双下肢胫骨前缘内侧有无凹陷性水肿。

当膝关节肿胀时检查浮髌现象,被检查者取平卧位,患肢伸直放松,检查者左手拇指和其他手指分别固定在肿胀膝关节上方两侧加压,压迫髌上囊,使关节腔内积液不能上下流动,然后用右手示指将髌骨连续向后方垂直按压数次,当按压时髌骨与关节面有碰触感,松开时有髌骨浮起感,此即为浮髌试验阳性。

检查者用手施压于被检查者大腿,嘱其做屈髋动作;检查者用手置于被检查者屈膝下肢的胫骨下方并施加压力,请被检查者对抗阻力做伸膝动作,检查肌力并两侧对比。放松下肢比较两侧肌张力。

检查者用左手在腘窝处托起下肢,使髋、膝关节稍屈,然后用叩诊锤叩击髌骨下方的股四头肌肌腱,观察小腿伸展动作,先查左侧,后查右侧膝腱反射,使被检查者髋、膝关节稍屈,下肢外旋外展位,检查者用左手使足掌背屈成直角,然后以叩诊锤叩击跟腱,观察足向跖面屈曲运动。同样方法检查右侧跟腱反射。检查髌阵挛时嘱被检查者伸直下肢,检查者以拇指与示指捏住髌骨上缘,用力向远端快速连续推动数次,后维持推力,阳性反应为股四头肌发生节律性收缩,使髌骨上、下移动。检查踝阵挛时嘱被检查者仰卧,髋、膝关节稍屈,检查者一手托住被检查者腘窝,一手持其足掌前端,突然用力使踝关节背屈,并维持之,阳性表现为腓肠肌和比目鱼肌发生节律性收缩,出现踝关节交替性屈伸动作。均同样先查左侧后查右侧。

检查者用竹签沿足底外侧缘,由后向前划至小趾跖趾关节处,再转向大拇趾侧,如拇趾缓缓背伸,其余四趾呈扇形展开,为 Babinski 征阳性。再检查右侧 Babinski 征。检查者用拇指和示指或示指和中指沿被检查者胫骨前缘用力由上向下滑压,阳性表现同 Babinski 征,称 Oppenheim 征阳性。将膝部稍抬起,检查者右手拇指及其他四指捏压腓肠肌,阳性表现同 Babinski 征,称 Gordon 征阳性。检查者用竹签在被检查者外踝下方足背外缘由后向前轻划,阳性表现均同 Babinski 征,称 Chaddock 征阳性,均先查左侧后查右侧。

(傅志君)

Chapter 7 Examinations of Spine, Extremities and Nervous System

Have the patient lie on his or her back and remove the quilt and the pillow. Place your hand behind the patient's neck and flex it until the chin touches the sternum. In patients with meningitis, there's neck pain and resistance to motion. There may also be flexion of the patient's hips and knees. This is called Brudzinski's nape of the neck sign. Another sign of meningeal irritation can be elicited while the patient lies on the back and you flex one of the patient's legs (left-side first) at the hip and the knee at 90 degrees. Then place your left hand on the knee, and right hand at the ankle. If pain and resistance is elicited as the knee is extended, a positive Kernig's sign is present. Normally, the knee can be extended to a degree greater than 135.

Have the patient sit down. Ask him or her to bend forward, backward, leftward and rightward from the neck and the waist to test the range of motion of the spine. An imaginary line drawn by your finger from the posterior occipital tuberosity should fall over the intergluteal cleft. Any lateral curvature is abnormal. Press each spinous process and the paravertebral muscles with your thumb for tenderness. Placing the palm of the left hand on the top of the patient's head and gently hitting it with the ulnar surface of the fist of your right hand elicit indirect percussion for tenderness. Note the location of the pain, as it is always related to the damage. Percuss each thoracolumbar spinous process with the reflex hammer for tenderness. Note the exact spinous process where pain is elicited, with a marker of C7's spinous process.

The abdominal superficial reflex is elicited by having the patient lie on his or her back. An application stick is quickly stroked in the direction of lateral to medial along the costal margins, toward the umbilicus and along the inguinal grooves. The result is a contraction of the abdominal muscles. Make a left-to-right comparison.

Now, inspect the skin, joints, fingers and nails of the upper extremities.

During inspection, deformities and liver palms should be noticed. The assessment of range of motion of specific joint is next to be assessed, e.g. extension, flexion, abduction, adduction and rotation of the shoulder; extension, flexion and rotation of the elbows; extension, flexion, supination and pronation of the wrists; extension and flexion of the finger joints. Any pain or resistance is abnormal. Place your right hand at the lateral aspect of the patient's left arm and supinate it. Test flexion strength by having the patient pull against your resistance. Place your right hand at the lateral aspect of the patient's left arm. Test extension strength by having the patient push against your resistance. Assess the muscle strength against resistance. Normal muscle power is grade 5. Test the right arm with the same method and compare with the left side. Ask the patient to grasp your extended index and middle fingers and to squeeze them as hard as possible. Compare the strength of both hands. Then ask the patient to relax and assess upper extremity tone.

The biceps tendon reflex is assessed by having the patient pronate the forearm midway between flexion and extension. The examiner should hold the patient's elbow and place the left thumb firmly on the biceps tendon. The hammer is then struck on the examiner's thumb. The examiner should observe for rapid contraction of the forearm followed by flexion at the elbow. The triceps tendon reflex is tested by flexing the patient's forearm at the elbow. The elbow should be midway between flexion and extension. Tap the triceps tendon above the insertion of the ulna's olecranon process just above the elbow. There should be a prompt contraction of the triceps with extension of the elbow. The brachioradialis tendon reflex is performed by having the patient's forearm in semiflexion and semipronation. The wrist should be drooping. The hammer should strike the styloid process of the radius. The examiner should observe for flexion at the elbow and simultaneous supination of the forearm. To elicit Hoffmann's sign, hold the patient's upper wrist with your left hand. Grasp the patient's middle finger between your right index finger and thumb, and lift up a bit to extend the wrist. With a sharp jerk, the middle finger is passively flexed and suddenly released. A positive response consists of adduction and flexion of the thumb as well as flexion of the other fingers. Test the right side in the same way.

For examining the lower extremities, expose the lower extremities. Inspect the skin and the veins. Deformities of the joints should be carefully noticed if present. Assess extension, flexion, abduction, adduction and rotation of the hips, extension, flexion and rotation of the knees, and dorsiflexion and plantar flexion of the ankles and the toes. Any pain or limit is abnormal. Press the shin areas to assess the pitting edema.

Testing for knee joint effusion is performed by

pressing the fluid out of the suprapatellar pouch down behind the patella. Have the patient lie on his or her back and relax the leg. Start above the superior margin of the patella and slide your left index finger and thumb firmly downward along the sides of the femur, milking the fluid into the space between the patella and femur. While you maintain pressure on the lateral margins of the patella, tap vertically on the patella with your right index finger. In the presence of floating patella phenomenon, a palpable tap will be felt, and the transmitted impulse will be felt by the fingers on either side of the patella.

Ask the patient to lift the knee towards his/her chest and pull it up as hard as possible. Put your hand against the patient's knee and try to overcome the pressure. Ask the patient to bend the knee. Put your hand on the shin area. Test the muscle strength by having the patient extend the knee against your hand. Relax and assess muscle tone of the lower extremity.

Perform the knee jerk by placing your left hand under the knee to flex the hip and the knee a little. Strike the quadriceps tendon below the patella with your reflex hammer. Observe the extension of the leg. Perform this on the left side first. The ankle jerk is elicited by having the patient flex the leg at the hip and the knee. The leg should be external rotated and abducted. The examiner places the left hand under the patient's foot to make ankle dorsiflexion at 90 degrees. The achilles tendon is struck with the reflex hammer. The result is plantar flexion at the ankle. With the leg straight take the patella with your thumb and finger and bring it briskly downwards; maintain it and the demonstration of clonus at the knee is a rhythmic contraction of the quadriceps may be noted, which makes the patella move up and down. Have the patient's hip and knee be flexed a little. The examiner should put one hand under the knee and the other hand under the foot. Make ankle dorsiflexion briskly; maintain the foot in that position. If a sudden rhythmic dorsiflexion and plantar flexion of the ankle occur due to the rhythmic contraction of the gastrocnemius and the soleus, ankle clonus is present. Always perform these tests on left side first.

Stroke the lateral aspect of the sole with an application stick from the heel to the ball of the foot and curved medially across the heads of the metatarsal bones. In the presence of Babinski's sign, there is dorsiflexion of the great toe, with fanning of the other toes. Oppenheim's sign is the same demonstration as Babinski's sign caused by thumb and index finger running down the medial aspect of the tibia. Gordon's sign has the same appearance as Babinski's sign, which is elicited by pinch the gastrocnemius with your fingers. When there is dorsiflexion of the great toe with fanning of the other toes on stroking the lateral aspect of the foot, Chaddock's sign is presented. Always start from the left side and continue to the right side.

Lin Haojie(林豪杰)　Zhong Chunjiu（钟春玖）

第八章 肛门、直肠、生殖器检查

根据病情需要应进行肛门、直肠、生殖器的检查,男医师检查女病人时,须有女医务人员在场。消除顾虑,保护隐私。

肛门、直肠检查常采取左侧卧位,观察肛门及周围皮肤,有无脓血、黏液、肛裂、外痔、瘘管、脓肿、脱肛及其他畸形等。做直肠指诊时,检查者右手示指戴指套或手套,并涂以润滑剂如液状石蜡等,先将探查的示指置于肛门外口轻轻按摩,等病人肛门括约肌放松后,探查示指再徐徐插入肛门直肠内,检查肛门括约肌的紧张度,以及直肠内壁有无触痛、包块,指套有无染血等。

一般不常规进行生殖器检查,如有必要,可请专科医师检查。检查外生殖器应充分暴露下身,检查有无畸形、异常分泌物、肿瘤、炎症等征象。

帮助患者擦拭被检查的部位并向患者提供纸巾,感谢被检查者的配合并道别。

(傅志君)

Chapter 8   Examination of Rectum, Anus and Genitalia

The rectum, anus and genitalia should be examined when necessary. If the patient is female, female medical workers should accompany their male medical workers to perform the rectal and genital examination. Ensure the privacy of the patient's and avoid uneasiness.

Ask the patient to take left lateral position, inspect his or her rectum and the peripheral skin. Notice the bloody pus, mucus, anal fissure, external hemorrhoids, fistula, abscess, prolapse or some other malformation if any. Lubricate the gloved fingers or the finger. Massage tightly the anus until the sphincter relaxed. Insert the tip of the index finger into the anal canal with gentle pressure and examine the tension of anal sphincter, notice any tenderness or masses. Examine the glove on withdrawal of your finger.

Genitalia are not examined in normal situations. Ask the specialist to examine genitalia if it is necessary. Ask the patient to expose completely, noticing any malformation, abnormal secretions, masses and inflammation.

Always wipe the checked part of the patient after examination and offer further tissues. Thank the patient for his or her cooperation and say good-bye.

Shi Hong（石虹）

第九章 住院病史

第一节 住院病史-1

姓名:王××
性别:男
年龄:45岁
婚姻:已婚
民族:汉
籍贯:上海
职业:工人
工作单位:上海××工厂
住址:上海市××路×号
入院时间:2006年×月×日
采史(记录)时间:2006年×月×日
供史者:患者本人(可靠)

主诉:

反复上腹部疼痛20年,加重2周,黑便2天。

现病史:

患者在既往20年中反复发作上腹疼痛。症状在秋末和早春加重,伴有恶心和反酸,进食后可缓解。6年前曾经解黑便,X线钡餐提示胃小弯后壁见直径1 cm龛影,黏膜向龛影集中,龛影的轮廓光滑。当时服用雷尼替丁以后好转。2周来,无明显诱因下上腹痛加重。昨天上午感到心悸和眩晕。解柏油样便,昨天3次,今天2次,总量约600 g。急诊查粪隐血++++。给予补液后立即收入消化科病房。

过去史:

病人既往无传染病史。因慢性扁桃体炎于5年前行扁桃体切除术。无食物和药物过敏史。预防接种规范。

系统回顾:

头部及器官:无视力减退、外耳道流脓、听力减退及长期流涕、鼻塞史。

呼吸系统:无咯血、慢性咳嗽及呼吸困难史。

循环系统:无下肢水肿、心前区疼痛、心悸及晕厥史。

消化系统:请见现病史。

内分泌系统:无烦渴、多尿及多饮,无震颤或多汗史。

血液系统:无皮下出血或贫血史。

泌尿生殖系统:无多尿、尿频、尿痛及显著的性欲下降史。

神经精神系统:无抽搐、感觉缺失、头痛及定向力障碍史。

运动系统:无关节肿痛、肌肉萎缩及营养不良史。

个人史:

出生、生长于上海,过去20年平均每天抽1

包烟,不喝酒。

婚育史:

25 岁结婚,妻子和儿子健康。

家族史:

父母健在。家族中无糖尿病、高血压、神经及精神病史。

体格检查:

体温37℃,脉搏86次/分,呼吸20次/分,血压120/80 mmHg。

一般情况:自主体位、发育良好、营养中等,表情自然,神志清晰,体检合作。

皮肤黏膜:无黄疸、皮疹、发绀和瘀斑,无肝掌或蜘蛛痣。

全身浅表淋巴结:未扪及肿大。

头部:头颅无畸形,头发黑色有光泽,无压痛。

眼:无眼睑水肿和下垂,结膜无充血,眼裂无增宽,瞳孔等大等圆,对光和调节反射存在,无眼球震颤、突眼或巩膜黄染,角膜透明。

耳:耳廓无异常,外耳道通畅无溢脓,乳突无压痛,听力正常。

鼻:外形正常,鼻腔无分泌物,鼻甲无肥大,鼻中隔无偏曲,鼻窦无压痛,鼻唇沟对称。

口:口唇红润,无发绀,牙齿无异常,舌苔薄白,口腔黏膜无瘀点和溃疡。咽无充血,扁桃体无肿大。

颈部:颈软,甲状腺无肿大,气管居中,无颈静脉怒张或异常搏动。

胸部:胸廓无畸形,胸骨无压痛。男性乳房无增生,无肿块或分泌物。

肺:

视诊:呼吸规则,胸式呼吸为主,呼吸运动度对称。

触诊:双侧语音震颤对称。

叩诊:肺叩诊清音,无浊音或过清音。

听诊:呼吸音清,无异常呼吸音和啰音。

心脏:

视诊:无心前区异常搏动。

触诊:心尖搏动位于第5肋间左锁骨中线内0.5 cm,无震颤。

叩诊:心脏大小正常,心脏相对浊音界如下表所示。

右界(cm)	肋间	左界(cm)
2.5	II	3
2.5	III	4
3	IV	7
	V	8.5

左锁骨中线距前正中线9 cm。

听诊:心音正常,无分裂。心率86次/分,律齐,无病理性杂音。

腹部:

视诊:平坦,无腹壁静脉曲张、肠型及胃肠蠕动波,腹式呼吸存在。

触诊:腹壁柔软,全腹无压痛、反跳痛,未及包块及肿大的脏器,Murphy征(-)。

叩诊:无移动性浊音,肝上界位于右锁骨中线第5肋间,肾区无叩痛。

听诊:肠鸣音活跃,10次/分,无血管杂音。

脊柱和四肢:下肢无水肿,无杵状指。脊柱和四肢关节无畸形,活动自如。

神经系统:生理反射存在,病理反射未引出。

泌尿生殖系统:正常男性外生殖器,无睾丸或阴囊水肿。

实验室检查:

血常规:

红细胞4.0×10^{12}/L,血红蛋白120 g/L,白细胞8.6×10^9/L,中性粒细胞73%,淋巴细胞24%,血小板167×10^9/L。

粪隐血:++++。

特殊检查:

胃镜:十二指肠球部前壁见0.5 cm×0.5 cm溃疡,基底部附血凝块,周围黏膜充血、水肿,尿素酶测试提示幽门螺杆菌阳性。

病史特点:

(1)男性,45岁,工人。

(2)反复上腹部疼痛20年,加重2周,黑便

2天。

(3) 体检:心率86次/分,血压120/80 mmHg。无黄疸,无肝掌、蜘蛛痣,腹软,无压痛,未扪及肿块及肿大脏器,肠鸣音活跃,双下肢无水肿。

(4) 血常规:红细胞 4.0×10^{12}/L,血红蛋白120 g/L,白细胞 8.6×10^9/L,中性粒细胞73%,淋巴细胞24%,血小板 167×10^9/L。粪隐血:++++。胃镜提示十二指肠球部前壁见 $0.5 \text{ cm} \times 0.5 \text{ cm}$ 溃疡,基底部附血凝块,周围黏膜充血、水肿。尿素酶测试提示幽门螺杆菌阳性。

初步诊断:

活动期十二指肠球部溃疡,幽门螺杆菌阳性。

诊疗计划:

(1) 奥美拉唑(20 mg)+克拉霉素(500 mg)+阿莫西林(1 000 mg),1天2次,服用1周。

(2) 1周后服用奥美拉唑每天1次,每次20 mg,以及达喜片每次1片,每天3次,共4周。

(3) 如果三联药物治疗后组织学或 ^{13}C 尿素酶呼吸试验提示幽门螺杆菌仍为阳性,选用四联治疗(铋剂+质子泵抑制剂+两种抗生素)作为二线治疗是必须的。

签名:×××

(石虹)

Chapter 9 Complete History

Complete History-1

Name: Wang × ×
Sex: Male
Age: 45
Marital status: Married
Nationality: Han
Birth place: Shanghai
Occupation: Worker
Job Unit: × ×Factory
Address: × ×Road, Shanghai
Date of admission: × × ,2006
Date of record: × × ,2006
Provider of medical history: patient himself (reliable)

Chief complaints:

Recurrent upper abdominal pain for 20 years, deteriorated for 2 weeks and black tarry stool for 2 days.

Present illness:

The patient often complained of upper abdominal pain in the past 20 years. The symptoms seemed to be worse during late fall and early spring with nausea and acid regurgitation and could be alleviated by food intake. He had one episode of tarry stool 6 years ago. Barium meal X-ray examination of stomach showed that a niche with 1 cm in diameter on the posterior wall of the lesser curvature, mucosal folds radiated into the crater and the niche outline was smooth. He took ranitidine and turned better. The upper abdominal pain deteriorated in the past 2 weeks without overt cause. Last morning he felt palpitation and dizziness. Then he had tarry stools three times yesterday and twice today, with the total amount of about 600 g. Occult blood tests showed + + + + of the stool in the emergency department. He was given fluid infusion and admitted into the gastroenterology ward immediately.

Past medical history:

No history of infectious disease. Tonsillectomy was performed for chronic tonsillitis before 5 years. He had no history of allergy to drugs or foods. Vaccinated regularly.

Review of systems:

Head: No poor vision. No ear purulent discharge. No hearing lose. No chronic running nose and nasal stuffiness.

Respiratory system: No history of hemoptysis, frequent cough or dyspnea.

Circulatory system: No edema in lower extremities. No precordial pain. No palpitation. No syncope.

Digestive system: Please refer to present illness.

Endocrine system: No polydipsia, polyuria or polyphagia. No tremor or excessive sweating.

Hematologic system: No history of subcutaneous bleeding or anemia.

Genitourinary system: No polyuria, urgency micturition, urodynia or decreased markedly sexual desire.

Neuropsychiatric system: No convulsion and anesthesia. No headaches. No abnormal orientation.

Locomotor system: No arthralgia, no muscular atrophies or dystrophies.

Personal history:

Born and grow up in Shanghai. He smokes an average of a packet of cigarettes daily for the past 20 years. No alcohol abuse.

Marital history:

He got married at the age of 25. His wife and

son are in good health.

Family history:

His parents are living and well. There was no family history of diabetes, hypertension or mental diseases.

Physical examination:

Temperature 37°C, Pulse 86/min, Respiration 20/min, Blood pressure 120/80 mmHg.

General appearance: Natural good erect posture. Well developed. Moderate nourished. Natural facial expression. Clear and cooperative in mentality.

Skin: No jaundice or rashes. No cyanosis and bruises. No liver palm or spider angioma.

Lymph nodes: Not enlarged.

Head: The shape of his head is normal. The hair is black and lustrous. No tenderness.

Eyes: No edema in eyelids, no ptosis, no conjunctival congestion. Width of palpebral fissures is normal. The pupils are round and equal, reactive well to light and accommodation. No nystagmus, exophthalmos or scleral jaundice. Cornea is transparent.

Ears: No abnormal pinnae. The external canals are clear without pus. No tenderness over the mastoids. Normal hearing in both ears.

Nose: The nose showed no deformity. No discharge. The turbinates are not hypertrophic. There is no deviation of the septum. No tenderness over the sinuses. The nasolabial grooves are equal bilaterally.

Mouth: Lips red. No cyanosis. All teeth are present and good. The tongue is thinly coated and is normal papillae. No petechiae and no ulcer in the mucosa. No injection on the pharynx. The tonsils are not enlarged.

Neck: Supple. The thyroid is not enlarged. The trachea is in the midline. No jugular vein prominence or abnormal pulsation.

Chest: Contour is normal. No sternum tenderness. The breasts are male without masses or discharge.

Lungs:

Inspection: The breathing is mainly thoracic in type. Degree of expansion is equal bilaterally.

Palpation: Tactile fremitus symmetrical on both sides.

Percussion: Lungs fields clear to percussion without dullness or hyperresonance.

Auscultation: Breath sounds are clear without pathological sounds or rales.

Heart:

Inspection: No abnormal pulsation.

Palpation: The PMI (point of maximum impulse) can be felt in 5th left intercostal space 0.5 cm inside of the mid clavicular line. No thrill.

Percussion: The heart percussed normal in size. Picture as follows:

right (cm)	intercostal	left (cm)
2.5	II	3
2.5	III	4
3	IV	7
	V	8.5

The left mid-clavicular line is 9 cm far from front midsternal line.

Auscultation: The heart sounds are strong and no splitting. A rate of 86/min. Cardiac rhythm is regular. No pathological murmurs.

Abdomen:

Inspection: Flat. No scar and no dilated vein seen. No gastral or intestinal pattern. No peristalsis. Abdominal respiration exists.

Palpation: Soft. No tenderness. No palpable masses or organomegaly. Murphy's sigh is negative.

Percussion: No shifting dullness. The upper border of the liver is in the 5th intercostal space inside of the right mid-clavicular line. Costovertebral angle tenderness is negative.

Auscultation: Bowel sounds active, 10/min. No vessel murmur.

Spine and extremities: No edema in lower extremities. No clubbed finger. No malformation or disorder of the movement of axial and appendicular bones.

Neural system: Physiological reflexes are present without pathological reflexes.

Genitourinary system: Normal adult external genitalia of man. No swelling testes or hydrocele.

Laboratory findings:

Blood routine test:
RBC $4.0 \times 10^{12}/L$, Hb $120 g/L$, WBC $8.6 \times 10^9/L$, neutrophil 73%, lymphocyte 24%, PLT $167 \times 10^9/L$.

Stool occult blood test: + + + +.

Special procedures:

Gastroscopy showed a 0.5 cm × 0.5 cm ulcer in the anterior wall of duodenal bulb with a blood clot in the base and marked edema and hyperemia in the circumference. The urease test indicated H. pylori were positive.

Features of case history:

(1) Male, 45 years old worker.

(2) Recurrent upper abdominal pain for 20 years, deteriorated for 2 weeks and black tarry stool for 2 days.

(3) P. E. Pulse: 86/min, Blood pressure:

120/80 mmHg. No jaundice. No liver palm or spider angioma. Abdomen: soft. No tenderness. No palpable masses or organomegaly. Bowel sounds active. No edema of lower limbs.

(4) Blood routine test: RBC 4.0×10^{12}/L, Hb 120g/L, WBC 8.6×10^9/L, neutrophil 73%, lymphocyte 24%, PLT 167×10^9/L. Stool occult blood test: + + + +. Gastroscopy showed a 0.5 cm ×0.5 cm ulcer in the anterior wall of duodenal bulb with a blood clot in the base and marked edema and hyperemia in the circumference. H. pylori positive.

Diagnosis:

Active duodenal bulb ulcer and positive H. pylori infection.

Diagnosis and treatment plans:

(1) Omeprazole (20 mg) + Clarithromycin (500 mg) + Amoxicillin (1 000 mg) bid for 1 week.

(2) Omeprazole 20 mg qd with Talcid #1 tid for 4 weeks.

(3) If histology or ^{13}C-urea breath test shows persistence of H. pylori 4 weeks after triple therapy, quadruple therapy (Bismuth + PPI + two antibiotics) as a second-line treatment is necessary.

Signature: × × ×
Shi Hong (石虹)

第二节　住院病史-2

姓名：李××
性别：男
年龄：38岁
婚姻：已婚
民族：汉
籍贯：上海
职业：出租车司机
工作单位：××公司
住址：上海市××路××号
入院时间：2003年×月×日
采史(记录)时间：2003年×月×日
供史者：患者本人(可靠)

主诉：

发热、咳痰伴左胸痛4天。

现病史：

患者于入院前4天沐浴时受凉，随后高热、寒战，头痛、咳嗽伴左侧胸痛。发病初期干咳，2天后出现白色黏痰，偶呈血性。发病后自觉胸痛、不适，故去医院就诊。血常规检查发现白细胞总数 $11.0 \times 10^9/L$，中性粒细胞85%，淋巴细胞11%。X线胸片显示左肺中野大片边缘模糊高密度斑片状影。给予头孢菌素Ⅳ 0.5 g，一天两次口服，以及止咳、退热等治疗，体温仍处于

38.5℃~40℃。

病程中患者轻度气急,精神状态、睡眠、食欲欠佳,无盗汗,大小便正常。

过去史：

病人既往无传染病史,预防接种规则,15岁时有阑尾切除术史。无食物和药物过敏史。

系统回顾：

头部及器官：无视力减退、外耳道流脓、听力减退及长期流涕、鼻塞史。

呼吸系统：无慢性咳嗽、发作性气喘、咯血及呼吸困难史。

循环系统：无下肢水肿、心前区疼痛、心悸及晕厥史。

消化系统：无恶心、呕吐、呕血、腹泻及血便史。

内分泌系统：无烦渴、多饮、多食及多尿史。

血液系统：无四肢瘀斑,以及鼻和牙龈出血史。

泌尿生殖系统：无尿频、尿急、排尿困难及血尿史。

神经精神系统：无抽搐、感觉缺失、头痛及定向力障碍史。

运动系统：无关节肿痛、肌肉萎缩及活动障碍史。

个人史：

出生于上海,少量抽烟,不喝酒。

婚育史：

25岁结婚,妻子和儿子健康。

家族史：

祖母死于肺癌。家族中无糖尿病、高血压、神经、精神病及脑卒中史。

体格检查：

体温39.5℃,脉搏96次/分,呼吸20次/分,血压120/80 mmHg。

一般情况：发育中等、营养良好,呼吸规则,稍气急。神志清晰,对答切题,体检合作。

全身浅表淋巴结：未扪及肿大。

皮肤黏膜：无黄疸、皮疹、出血点及发绀。

头部及器官：头颅无畸形,无压痛,头发无缺失。

眼：无眼睑水肿和下垂,结膜无充血,眼裂无增宽,巩膜无黄染,角膜透明,瞳孔大小和形态正常,眼球无突出。

耳：外耳道无畸形,乳突无压痛,听力正常。

鼻：通畅,外形正常。鼻中隔无偏曲,鼻腔无分泌物,鼻窦无压痛。

口：无口唇疱疹,无牙龈溢脓和出血,无龋齿和义齿,伸舌居中,扁桃体不大。

颈部：颈软,气管居中,甲状腺无肿大,无颈静脉怒张。

胸部：胸廓无畸形,胸骨无压痛。

肺：

视诊：呼吸规则，呼吸运动对称。

触诊：左中肺语音震颤增强。

叩诊：左肺叩诊浊音。右肺下界位于肩胛线第9肋间、腋中线第7肋间、锁骨中线第5肋间，肺下界移动度5 cm。

听诊：左肺语音共振增强，左腋下及左前胸可闻及湿啰音，右肺呼吸音清。

心脏：

视诊：心尖搏动无异常，未见心前区隆起。

触诊：心尖搏动位于第5肋间左锁骨中线内1 cm，搏动范围直径约1.5 cm。

叩诊：心脏相对浊音界如下表所示。

右界(cm)	肋间	左界(cm)
2.5	Ⅱ	3
2.5	Ⅲ	4
3	Ⅳ	7
	Ⅴ	8.5

锁骨中线距前正中线9 cm。

听诊：心率：96次/分，律齐，心音正常，无杂音及心包摩擦音。

周围血管征：无水冲脉，枪击音及毛细血管搏动。

腹部：

视诊：平坦，无腹壁静脉曲张、肠型及蠕动波，腹式呼吸存在。

触诊：腹壁柔软，全腹无压痛、反跳痛，未及包块。肝、脾肋下未及，未触及包块及压痛，胆囊未及，Murphy 征(-)，肾未及，输尿管点无压痛。

叩诊：无移动性浊音，肝上界位于右锁骨中线第 5 肋间，肾区无叩痛。

听诊：肠鸣音 5 次/分，无振水音及血管杂音。

脊柱和四肢：脊柱无畸形，活动自如。下肢无水肿，无杵状指。四肢关节无红肿及畸形，活动正常。

神经反射：双侧腹壁反射、膝腱反射正常。Babinski 征、Kernig 征、Hoffmann 征均(-)。

肛门、直肠、外生殖器：未查。

实验室检查：

血常规：

白细胞总数 11.0×10^9/L，中性粒细胞 85%，淋巴细胞 11%。

血沉：34 mm/h。

尿常规：(-)。

粪常规：(-)。

特殊检查：

心电图：正常。

X 线胸片：左肺中野大片边缘模糊高密度斑片状影。

痰培养：大量肺炎链球菌生长，青霉素中介耐药。

病史特点:

(1) 李××,男性,38岁。

(2) 受凉后发热、咳痰伴左胸痛4天入院。

(3) 体检:体温39.5℃,左肺叩诊浊音,语音震颤增强,左腋下及左前胸可闻及湿啰音。

(4) X线胸片:左肺中野大片边缘模糊高密度斑片状影。痰培养:大量肺炎链球菌生长,青霉素中介耐药。血常规:白细胞总数 11.0 × 10^9/L,中性粒细胞85%。

初步诊断:

左侧肺炎链球菌肺炎。

诊疗计划:

(1) 动脉血气分析。

(2) 氧疗。

(3) 头孢曲松钠2 g溶于5% GNS 250 ml,静滴,1天1次。

(4) 沐舒坦60 mg p.o,1天2次。

(5) 对症治疗,如:退热治疗。

(6) 卧床休息,多饮水。

签名:×××

(王葆青)

Complete History-2

Name: Li × ×
Sex: Male
Age: 38
Marital status: Married
Nationality: Han
Birth place: Shanghai
Occupation: Taxi driver
Job Unit: × ×Co.
Address: Rm × × ×Rd., Shanghai
Investigate (record) Date: × ×, 2003
Admission date: 9:30 a.m. × ×, 2003
Provider: Patient(reliable)

Chief complaints:

Onset fever, productive cough, and chest pain for 4 days.

Present illness:

The patient got a cold in a bath four days before admission. He experienced shiver, high fever, headache and cough. At the beginning of the illness the cough was dry, but two days later the cough was productive. The sputum was white, occasionally with blood streaking. He complained of chest pain and general discomfort. So, he went to see a doctor. His blood routine examination showed the total leucocyte count was 11.0×10^9/L with neutrophil 85%, lymph 11%. His radiogram of chest showed panlobular patchy intensive shadow in the middle area of left lung. He was treated with Cephalosporin Ⅳ 0.5 g p.o. twice a day, cough drops, and antifebrile which turned out to be ineffective. He felt better of his cough, but the fever still stayed between 38.5℃ ~ 40℃.

He was in a moderate distress. His mental state, appetite, and sleeping patterns were influenced. He denied night sweat. There was no change in bowel habit or urination.

Past medical history:

No history of infectious diseases. Vaccinated regularly. He had an appendectomy at 15 years old. He is not allergic to any drugs and foods.

Review of systems:

Head: No poor vision. No ear purulent discharge. No hearing lose. No chronic running nose and nasal stuffiness.

Respiratory system: No chronic cough and in a fit of breathlessness. No hemoptysis. No dyspnea.

Circulatory system: No edema in lower extremities. No precordial pain. No palpitation. No syncope.

Digestive system: No vomiting and diarrhea. No hematemesis and bloody stool.

Endocrine system: No polydipsia or polyuria or polyphagia.

Hematologic system: No bruises on limbs. No nasal hemorrhage or gingival bleeding.

Genito-urinary system: No dysuria. No urinary frequency. No precipitant urination or urodynia. No hematuria.

Neuropsychiatric system: No convulsion and anesthesia. No headaches. No abnormal orientation.

Locomotor system: No muscular atrophies or dystrophies.

Personal history:

Born and grow up in Shanghai. Smokes occasionally. No alcohol abuse.

Marital history:

He was married at 25 years old. His wife and a boy are in good health.

Family history:

Maternal grandmother died of lung cancer. There was no family history of diabctes、hypertension and stroke. No family history of nervous or mental diseases.

Physical examination:

Temperature 39.5℃, Pulse 96/min. Respirations 20/min, Blood pressure 120/80 mmHg.

General appearance: The patient was in moderate distress, well developed and nourished. Regular respirations.

Lymph nodes: Not enlarged.

Skin: No jaundice or rashes. No cyanosis and bruises.

Head: skull and scalp normal. No tenderness. No loss of hair.

Eyes: No edema in eyelids, ptosis, no conjunctival injection. Width of palpebral fissures is normal. No jaundice. Pupils' size and shape is normal. Corneal is clear. No exophthalmos.

Ears: Auditory acuity is excellent. No ear purulent discharge.

Nose: Shape is normal. No obstruction. No deviation of nasal septum.

Mouth: No lips herpes. No cyanosis. No gums pyorrhea and bleeding. No tongue deviation. No caries and false teeth. Tonsils not enlarged.

Neck: His neck is soft. Trachea in the midline. No thyroid abnormality was found. Neck vein was not distended.

Chest: Contour is normal. No sternum tenderness.

Lungs:

Inspection: Respiration regular. Degree of expansion is symmetry.

Palpation: Tactile fremitus obvious in the left lung.

Percussion: Left lung dull to percussion. The lower border of right lung is in 9th, 7th, 5th intercostal space in scapular line, midaxillary line, midclavicular line respectively. The respiratory excursion of the lower lung margins is 5 cm.

Auscultation: Vocal fremitus obvious. Rales clear to auscultation in the left axillary and posterior area. The sounds in right lung are clear.

Heart:

Inspection: No abnormal pulsation or retraction.

Palpation: The apex beat can be felt in the 5th intercostal space 1 cm inside of the left mid-clavicular line.

Percussion: The border of cardiac is not enlarged.

Auscultation: The heart sounds were of good quality and the rhythm was regular. Heart rate: 96/min. No Bruits.

right(cm)	intercostal	left(cm)
2.5	II	3
2.5	III	4
3	IV	7
	V	8.5

The mid-clavicular line is 9 cm far from midsternal line.

Peripheral artery sign: No water hammer pulse, pistol shot sound or capillary pulsation sign.

Abdomen:

Inspection: Flat. No dilated veins. No gastral or intestinal pattern. No peristalsis. Abdominal respiration exists.

Palpation: Soft. Liver and spleen was not enlarged. No organomegaly or masses. No tenderness. Murphy's sign is negative.

Percussion: No shifting dullness. The upper border of the liver is in the 5th intercostal space inside of the right mid-clavicular line. Renal region: No percussion pain.

Auscultation: Bowel sound clear. 5ppm. No vessel murmur.

Spine and extremities: No edema in lower extremities. No clubbed finger. No disorder of the movement of axial and appendicular bones.

Reflex: Symmetrical, equal without pathological responses. Babinski sign and Kernig sign and

Hoffmann sign are all negative.

Genitalia: Not examined.

Laboratory findings:

Peripheral blood routine:

WBC count 11.0 ×10^9/L, Neutrophil 85%, Lymphocyte 11%

ESR: 34 mm/h

Urine routine: (−)

Stool routine: (−)

Special procedures:

EKG: Normal.

Chest X-ray: Poorly defined panlobular patchy intensive shadow in the middle area of left lung.

Culture of sputum: Lots of Streptococcus pneumonia was present. Intermediate resistance to Penicillin G.

Features of case history:

(1) Male, 38 years old.

(2) Onset fever, productive cough, and right chest pain for 4 days.

(3) P. E: Temperature: 39.5℃. Left lung dull to percussion. Vocal fremitus obvious. Rales clear to auscultation in the left axillary and posterior area.

(4) Chest X-ray: poorly defined panlobular

patchy intensive shadow in the middle area of left lung. Culture of sputum: Lots of Streptococcus pneumoniae was present. Peripheral blood routine: WBC count 11.0 ×10^9/L, Neutrophil 85%.

Diagnosis:

Pneumococcal pneumonia in the left lobe.

Diagnosis and treatment plans:

(1) Arterial blood gas analysis.

(2) Oxygen therapy.

(3) Ceftriaxone Sodium 2 g dissolved into 5% GNS 250 ml, ivgtt qd.

(4) Mucosolvan 60 mg p.o. bid.

(5) Allopathy, e.g. defervescence.

(6) Bed rest and drinking more water.

Signature: × × ×
Wang Baoqing（王葆青）

附录1 《规范体格检查及病史书写双语手册》中文—英文单词表

(按汉语拼音顺序)

A

凹陷性水肿	pitting edema

B

斑点	spot
板指	feeling finger
半卧位	semireclining position
背屈	dorsiflexion
鼻窦	paranasal sinus
鼻前庭	nasal vestibule
鼻腔	nasal cavity
鼻中隔	nasal septum
搏动	pulsation
边界	edge
扁桃体	tonsillar
表面	surface
表面光滑	lubricous surface

C

侧弯	lateral curvature
充血	congestion, engorgement
传导	conduction

D

胆囊	gall bladder
抵抗感	resistance

E

额窦	frontal sinus
耳后淋巴结	post-auricular node
耳前淋巴结	preauricular node

F

范围,幅度	range
腓肠肌	gastrocnemius
肺尖	apex of lung
分泌物	secretion
浮髌现象	floating patella phenomenon
腹壁	abdominal wall
腹壁浅反射	abdominal superficial reflex
腹股沟淋巴结	groin lymph node
腹直肌	rectus abdominis muscle

G

肝掌	liver palm
肛门	anus
肛门括约肌	anal sphincter
跟腱	achilles tendon
肱骨上髁	epicondyle of the humerus
鼓音区	tympanic area
关节	joint
关节积液	knee joint effusion
规则	regular
腘窝淋巴结	popliteal lymph node

H

横径	transverse diameter
颌下淋巴结	submaxillary node
红白交替现象,毛细血管搏动征	"red-white commutation" phenomenon
呼气	expiration
踝反射	ankle jerk
踝阵挛	ankle clonus
滑车上淋巴结	supratrochlear lymph node
后胸	metathorax

J

畸形	deformity, malformation
颊黏膜	buccal mucosa
甲状软骨	thyroid cartilage
甲状腺颊部	isthmus of thyroid
减弱	weaken
角膜反射	corneal reflex
节律	rhythm
紧张度	tense
颈	neck
颈动脉	carotid artery
颈动脉杂音	carotid bruit
颈静脉	jugular vein
颈深淋巴结	deep cervical node
静脉曲张	varicose vein, varicosity

K

叩诊槌	plexor
扩张度	expandability

L

淋巴结	lymph node
隆起	hunch
瘘管	fistula

M

麦氏征	Murphy sign

N

内收	adduction
粘连	adhesion
脓血	bloody pus
脓肿	abscess

P

平稳	stable

Q

气管	trachea
髂前上棘	anterior superior iliac spine
前后径	anteroposterior diameter
前肾点	anterior kidney point
浅表	superficial
浅表淋巴结	superficial lymph node
强度	intensity
屈曲	extension

R

乳突淋巴结	mastoid node
融合	fusion

热,灼热感	cauma
蠕动波	peristalsis
乳腺增生	mammoplasia

S

筛窦	ethmoid sinus
上方	superior
上颌骨	maxillae
上输尿管点	upper ureter point
上肢	upper extremities
上肢肌张力	upper extremity tone
肾下垂	nephroptosia
生殖器	genitalia
示指	index finger
收缩	contraction
收缩期	systole
手电筒	flashlight
舒张期	diastole
双手触诊法	bimanual method
损伤	lesion
伸展	flexion

T

听诊	auscultation
听诊器	stethoscope
痛	pain
头部	head

突出	protrusion
臀间裂	intergluteal cleft
脱垂	prolapse
抬举性搏动	palpable heave
体温计	clinical thermometer

W

外展	abduction
外痔	external hemorrhoid
尾部	tail
胃肠型	gastrointestinal pattern
胃扩张	gastric dilatation

X

吸气	inspiration
下方	inferior
下肢	lower extremity
下肢肌张力	lower extremity tone
消毒棉签	disinfectant cotton swab
小鱼际	hypothenar
心前区	precordium
性质	quality
胸部	thorax
胸廓	thoracic cage
胸锁关节	sternoclavicular joint
胸椎棘突	thoracolumbar spinous
旋后	supination

旋前	pronation
旋转	rotation
悬雍垂	uvula
血压计	sphygmomanometer

Y

压舌板	spatula
咽后壁	posterior pharynx
炎症	inflammation
眼睑下垂	dropping of eyelids
眼球运动障碍	malfunction of eye movement
仰卧位	supine position
腋窝淋巴结	axillary node
一般检查	general examination
一致	consistent
异常搏动	pathologic impulse
异常分泌物	abnormal secretion
溢脓	purulence
硬度	hardness
硬结	induration
幽门梗阻	pyloric obstruction
游走肾	floating kidney

Z

展开	fanning
脂肪充实度	flat enrichment

直肠	rectum
直尺	ruler
质地	texture
中输尿管点	middle ureter point
肿大,肿胀	swelling
肿块	lump
肘	elbow
左侧卧位	left lateral position

徐蓓莉(Xu Beili)　石虹(Shi Hong)

附录2 《规范体格检查及病史书写双语手册》英文—中文单词表

(按英文字母顺序)

A

abdominal superficial reflex	腹壁浅反射
abdominal wall	腹壁
abduction	外展
abnormal secretion	异常分泌物
abscess	脓肿
achilles tendon	跟腱
adduction	内收
adhesion	粘连
anal sphincter	肛门括约肌
ankle clonus	踝阵挛
ankle jerk	踝反射
anterior kidney point	前肾点
anterior superior iliac spine	髂前上棘
anteroposterior diameter	前后径
anus	肛门
apex of lung	肺尖

auscultation	听诊
axillary node	腋窝淋巴结

B

Babinski's sign	巴彬斯基征
bimanual method	双手触诊法
bloody pus	脓血
buccal mucosa	颊黏膜

C

carotid artery	颈动脉
carotid bruit	颈动脉杂音
cauma	热,灼热感
clinical thermometer	体温计
congestion	充血
consistent	一致
contraction	收缩
corneal reflex	角膜反射

D

deep cervical node	颈深淋巴结
deformity	畸形
diastole	舒张期
disinfectant cotton swab	消毒棉签
dorsiflexion	背屈
dropping of eyelids	眼睑下垂

E

edge	边界
elbow	肘
engorgement	充血
epicondyle of the humerus	肱骨上髁
ethmoid sinus	筛窦
expandability	扩张度
expiration	呼气
extension	屈曲
external hemorrhoid	外痔

F

fanning	展开
feeling finger	板指
fistula	瘘管
flashlight	手电筒
flat enrichment	脂肪充实度
flexion	伸展
floating kidney	游走肾
floating patella phenomenon	浮髌现象
frontal sinus	额窦
fusion	融合

G

gall bladder	胆囊
gastric dilatation	胃扩张
gastrocnemius	腓肠肌
gastrointestinal pattern	胃肠型
general examination	一般检查
genitalia	生殖器
Gordon's sign	戈登征
groin lymph node	腹股沟淋巴结

H

hardness	硬度
head	头部
hunch	隆起
hypothenar	小鱼际

I

index finger	示指
induration	硬结
inferior	下方
inflammation	炎症
intensity	强度
isthmus of thyroid	甲状腺颊部

J

joint	关节
jugular vein	颈静脉

K

Kernig's sign	凯尔尼格征
knee joint effusion	关节积液

L

lateral curvature	侧弯
left lateral position	左侧卧位
lesion	损伤
liver palm	肝掌
lower extremity	下肢
lower extremity tone	下肢肌张力
lubricous surface	表面光滑
lump	肿块
lymph node	淋巴结

M

malformation	畸形
malfunction of eye movement	眼球运动障碍
mammoplasia	乳腺增生
mastoid node	乳突淋巴结
maxillae	上颌骨

metathorax	后胸
middle ureter point	中输尿管点
Murphy sign	麦氏征

N

nasal cavity	鼻腔
nasal septum	鼻中隔
nasal vestibule	鼻前庭
neck	颈
nephroptosia	肾下垂

P

pain	痛
palpable heave	抬举性搏动
paranasal sinus	鼻窦
pathologic impulse	异常搏动
peristalsis	蠕动波
pitting edema	凹陷性水肿
plexor	叩诊槌
popliteal lymph node	腘窝淋巴结
post-auricular node	耳后淋巴结
posterior pharynx	咽后壁
preauricular node	耳前淋巴结
precordium	心前区
prolapse	脱垂
pronation	旋前
protrusion	突出

pulsation	搏动
purulence	溢脓
pyloric obstruction	幽门梗阻

Q

quality	性质

R

range	范围,幅度
rectum	直肠
rectus abdominis muscle	腹直肌
"red-white commutation" phenomenon	红白交替现象,毛细血管搏动征
regular	规则
resistance	抵抗感
rhythm	节律
rotation	旋转
ruler	直尺

S

secretion	分泌物
semireclining position	半卧位
spatula	压舌板
sphygmomanometer	血压计
spot	斑点
stable	平稳
sternoclavicular joint	胸锁关节

stethoscope	听诊器
submaxillary node	颌下淋巴结
superficial lymph node	浅表淋巴结
superior	上方
supratrochlear lymph node	滑车上淋巴结
supination	旋后
supine position	仰卧位
surface	表面
swelling	肿大,肿胀
systole	收缩期

T

tail	尾部
tense	紧张度
texture	质地
thoracic cage	胸廓
thoracolumbar spinous process	胸椎棘突
thorax	胸部
thyroid cartilage	甲状软骨
tonsillar	扁桃体
trachea	气管
transverse diameter	横径
tympanic area	鼓音区

U

upper extremities	上肢

upper extremity tone	上肢肌张力
upper ureter point	上输尿管点
uvula	悬雍垂

V

varicose vein, varicosity	静脉曲张

W

weaken	减弱

徐蓓莉(Xu Beili)　　石虹(Shi Hong)

附录3 《临床诊断学》中文—英文单词表

(按汉语拼音顺序)

A

艾迪生病	Addison's disease
鞍鼻	saddle nose
昂白征	Romberg's sign
奥本海姆征	Oppenheim's sign

B

巴彬斯基征	Babinski's sign
白斑	leukoplakia
白癜	vitiligo
白化病	albinismus
瘢痕	scar
斑丘疹	maculopapular
斑疹	maculae
板状腹	board-like rigidity
包茎	phimosis
包块	mass
包皮	prepuce
包皮垢	smegma

包皮过长	prepuce redundant
爆裂音	crackle
被动抬腿动作	passive leg raising maneuver
被动体位	passive position
奔马律	gallop rhythm
鼻出血	epistaxis
鼻窦	nasal sinus
鼻咽	nasal pharynx
闭孔内肌试验	obturator maneuver
扁平胸	flat chest
变形颅	deforming skull
表情	expression
髌阵挛	patella clonus
病危面容	critical facies
波动感	fluctuation
勃起	erection
不良	poorly
步态	gait
部位	location
不自主运动	abnormal movements
布鲁津斯基征	Brudzinski's sign

C

苍白	pallor
草莓舌	strawberry tongue
层流	laminar flow
查多克征	Chaddock's sign

长颅	delichocephalia
肠鸣音	bowel sound
肠型	intestinal pattern
超力型,矮胖型	sthenic type
潮式呼吸	tidal breathing
痴呆	dementia
迟脉	tardus pulse
尺压试验	ruler pressing test
冲击触诊法	ballottement
重叠性奔马律	summation gallop
抽搐	tics
杵状指(趾)	acropachy
触发活动	triggered activity
触觉语颤	tactile fremitus
处女膜	hymen
触诊	palpation
粗湿啰音	coarse rales
错觉	illusion

D

大小	size
大阴唇	labium majus
呆小病	cretinism
单纯雀斑样痣	lentigo simplex
等张握力运动	isometric hand grip
低调干啰音	sonorous rhonchi
低血压	hypotension

抵抗	oppositional paratonia
第二心音	second heart sound
第三心音	third heart sound
第四心音	fourth heart sound
地图舌	geographic tongue
第一心音	first heart sound
点头运动	deMusset's sign
定向力	orientation
定向障碍	disorientation
动态血压监测	ambulatory blood pressure measurement, ABPM
动眼神经	oculomotor n.
Valsalva 动作	Valsalva maneuver
杜加斯征	Dugas' sign
杜柔双重音	Duroziez's sign
端坐呼吸	orthopnea
短暂阻断动脉血流	transient arterial occlusion
对称性	symmetry

E

额外心音	extra cardiac sound
恶性黑色素瘤	malignant melanoma
恶病质	cachexia
耳廓	auricle
耳聋	deafness
耳蜗神经	cochlear n.
耳语音增强	whispered pectoriloquy

二尖瓣反流	mitral regurgitation
二尖瓣关闭不全	mitral insufficiency
二尖瓣面容	mitral facies
二尖瓣脱垂综合征	mitral valve prolapse syndrome
二尖瓣狭窄	mitral stenosis
二联律	bigeminal beats

F

发绀	cyanosis
发红	redness
发射	reflex
发育	development
反常分裂	paradoxical splitting
反跳痛	rebound tenderness
方颅	squared skull
房性奔马律	atrial gallop
肥胖	obesity
肺不张	atelectasis
肺动脉瓣区	pulmonary valve area
肺动脉喀喇音	pulmonary ejection click
肺泡呼吸音	vesicular breath sound
肺气肿	pulmonary emphysema
肺实变	consolidation of lung
肺循环淤血	pulmonary congestion
浮肋	free ribs
附睾	epididymis

附睾囊肿	epididymal cyst
附加音	adventitious sound
副神经	spinal accessory n.
复视	diplopia
负性心尖搏动	inward impulse
腹白线	linea alba
腹壁反射	abdominal reflexes
腹部凹陷	abdominal concavity
腹部膨隆	abdominal protuberance
腹部肿块	abdominal mass
腹股沟韧带	inguinal ligament
腹膜刺激征	peritoneal irritation sign
腹上角	upper abdominal angle
腹式呼吸	diaphragmatic respiration
腹水	ascites
腹直肌外缘	lateral border of rectus muscles
腹中线	midabdominal line

G

肝病面容	hepatic facies
肝大	hepatomegaly
肝豆状核变性	hepatolenticular degeneration
肝颈静脉回流征	hepatojugular reflux
肝震颤	liver thrill
感觉	sensation
感觉过敏	hyperesthesia

感觉减退	hypoesthesia
感觉性失语	sensory aphasia
感觉障碍	disorders of sensation
感知综合障碍	psychosensory disturbance
干啰音	dry rales /rhonchi
肛管	anal canal
肛裂	anal fissure
肛瘘	hedrosyrinx
高调干啰音	sibilant rhonchi
睾丸	testis
高血压	hypertension
戈登征	Gordon's sign
跟腱反射	achilles reflex
跟臀试验	Ely test
跟膝胫试验	heel-knee-tibia test
肱二头肌反射	biceps reflex
宫颈	cervix uteri
功能性杂音	functional murmur
肱三头肌反射	triceps reflex
宫体	corpus uteri
巩膜	sclera
共济失调	ataxia
共济失调步态	ataxic gait
佝偻病串珠	rachitic rosary
佝偻病胸	rachitic chest
钩指触诊	hook technique
钩指触诊法	hook method

构音困难	dysphonia
咕噜声	gurgling sound
骨导	bone conduction
鼓音	tympany
固定分裂	fixed splitting
关节觉	joint position sense
光滑舌	smooth tongue
过清音	hyperresonance

H

黑棘皮病	acanthosis nigricans
黑色素	melanin
虹膜	iris
喉	larynx
喉咽	laryngeal pharynx
后除极	after depolarization
后跟试验	heel jar test
后正中线	posterior midline
呼吸	respiration
呼吸过缓	bradypnea
呼吸过速	tachypnea
呼吸节律和幅度	respiratory rhythm and range
呼吸困难	dyspnea
呼吸频率	respiratory frequency
呼吸深度	respiratory depth
呼吸运动	breathing movement
胡萝卜素	carotene

滑车神经	trochlear n.
踝阵挛	ankle clonus
幻觉	hallucination
慌张步态	festinating gait
黄疸	jaundice
黄褐斑	chloasma
黄染	stained yellow
会阴	perineum
昏迷	coma
昏睡	stupor
活动度	mobility
霍夫曼征	Hoffmann's sign

J

基底节	basal ganglion
机器声样杂音	machinery murmur, Gibson murmur
肌束颤动	fasciculation
肌纤维颤搐	myokymia
鸡胸	keeled chest, pigeon chest
肌张力	muscle tone
肌阵挛	myoclonus
集合反射	convergency reflex
脊柱侧凸	scoliosis
脊柱后凸	kyphosis
脊柱棘突	spinous process
脊柱前凸	lordosis

记忆	memory
继发性高血压,症状性高血压	secondary hypertension
家族性进行性色素过度沉着症	familial progressive hyper-pigmantation
甲状腺	thyroid
甲状腺功能亢进	hyperthyroidism
尖腹	apical belly
肩胛骨	scapula
肩胛间区	interscapular region
肩胛区	scapular region
肩胛上区	suprascapular region
肩胛下区	infrascapular region
肩胛线	scapular line
间接叩诊	mediate percussion
间接叩诊法	indirect percussion
间接听诊法	indirect auscultation
尖颅	oxycephaly
尖颅并指(趾)畸形	acro-cephalosyndactylia
间歇性跛行	intermittent claudication
剪刀式步态	scissors gait
睑内翻	entropion
检眼镜	ophthalmoscope
剑突	xiphoid process
交替脉	pulsus alternans
角弓反张位	opisthotonos position

角膜	cornea
角膜反射	corneal reflex
结肠充气试验	Rovsing's test
结节性红斑	erythema nodosum
结膜	conjunctiva
近反射	near reflex
精囊	seminal vesicle
精神障碍	mental disorder
精神状态	mental status
精索	spermatic cord
精索积液	hydrocele of cord
精子囊肿	spermatocele
颈动脉搏动增强	visible pulsation of carotid artery, Corrigan's sign
颈静脉充盈	jugular vein distension
痉挛	spasm
静脉	vein
静止性震颤	static tremor
酒渣鼻	rosacea
橘皮	orange peel
巨大 a 波	cannon wave, cannon "a" wave
巨颅	large skull

K

开瓣音	opening snap
凯尔尼格征	Kernig's sign

克莱恩费特综合征	Klinefelter syndrome
空瓮音	amphorophony
口	mouth
口咽	oral pharynx
叩诊	percussion
叩诊音	percussion sound
苦笑面容	sardonic feature
库欣综合征	Cushing syndrome
跨阈步态	steppage gait
髋关节承重功能试验	Trendelenburg test
溃疡	ulcer

L

老年环	arcus senilis
肋膈窦	sinus phrenicocostalis
肋膈沟	Harrison's groove
肋弓下缘	costal margin
肋骨	rib
肋脊角	costovertebral angle
肋间隙	intercostal space
理想体重	ideal body weight
连续性杂音	continuous murmur
两点辨别感觉	two-point tactile discrimination
裂纹舌	wrinkled tongue
漏斗胸	funnel chest

卵巢	ovary
轮替动作	alternate motion
啰音	rales
落日现象	setting sun phenomenon

M

麻痹性斜视	paralytic squint
麻疹黏膜斑	Koplik spot
脉搏	pulse
脉搏短绌,短绌脉	pulse deficit
麦氏点,阑尾点	McBurney point
脉压	pulse pressure, PP
满月面容	moon facies
毛发	hair
毛舌	hairy tongue
毛细血管搏动征	capillary pulsation sign
玫瑰疹	roseola
蒙古斑	Mongolian spot
糜烂	erosion
迷走神经	vagus n.
面容	facial features
面神经	facial n.
命名性失语	nominal aphasia
摩擦音	friction rubs

N

脑神经	cranial n.

逆分裂	reversed splitting
黏液性水肿	myxedema
年龄	age
捻发音	crepitus
尿道口	urethral meatus
牛肉舌	beefy tongue
脓疱	pustule

P

蹒跚步态	waddling gait
疱疹	bleb
喷射音	ejection sound
脾大	splenomegaly
皮肤脱屑	desquamation
皮肤血管瘤	cutaneous hemangiomas
皮下出血	subcutaneous bleeding
皮下结节	subcutaneous nodules
皮下气肿	subcutaneous emphysema
皮褶厚度	skinfold thickness
皮疹	skin eruption

Q

期前收缩	premature contraction
脐	umbilicus
脐部	umbilical region
奇脉	paradoxical pulse, pulsus paradoxus

气导	air conduction
气腹	pneumoperitoneum
气胸	pneumothorax
器质性杂音	organic murmur
髂前上棘	anterior superior iliac spine
牵涉痛	referred pain
牵涉性触痛	referred tenderness
荨麻疹	urticaria
前列腺	prostate gland
前庭大腺	major vestibular grands
前正中线	anterior midline
浅部触诊法	light palpation
枪击音	pistol shot
强迫蹲位	compulsive squatting
强迫体位	compulsive position
强迫停立位	forced standing position
清音	resonance
情感	emotion
情感反应	affect
丘疹	papules
全身体格检查	complete physical examination
全收缩期杂音	holosystolic murmur, pansystolic murmur
雀斑	freckle

R

桡反射	radial periosteal
任内试验	Rinne test, RT
揉面感	dough kneading sensation
蠕动波	peristalsis
乳房	breast
乳头	nipple
乳头乳晕角化过度症	hyperkeratosis of the nipple and areola
乳突	mastoid
乳晕	areola of breast
软下疳	chancroid
瑞-舒测试法	Wright-Schober test

S

腮腺	parotid gland
三凹征	three depressions sign
三叉神经	trigeminal n.
三尖瓣区	tricuspid valve area
三联律	trigeminal beats
搔刮试验	scratch test
色觉	color sensation
色素沉着	pigmentation
色素沉着-息肉综合征	Peutz Jeghers syndrome
筛查	screening examination

伤寒面容	typhoid facies
上臂周径	arm circumference
上腹部	epigastric region
上睑下垂	ptosis
舌	tongue
舌下神经	hypoglossal n.
舌咽神经	glossopharyngeal n.
深部触诊法	deep palpation
深部滑行触诊法	deep slipping palpation
深呼吸试验	cycled respiration test
深压触诊法	deep press palpation
肾病面容	nephritic facies
肾上腺皮质功能减退症	Addison disease
生理性分裂	physiologic splitting
生命征	vital sign
声嘶	hoarseness
失读症	alexia
湿啰音	moist rale
施瓦巴赫试验	Schwabach test, ST
湿度	moisture
失写症	agraphia
失用症	apraxia
失语	aphasia
实体辨别觉	stereognosis
实音	flatness
匙状指	koilonychia

视力	visual acuity
视力障碍	visual disorder
视神经	optic n.
室性奔马律	ventricular gallop
视野	visual fields
视诊	inspection
嗜睡	somnolence
收缩期喀喇音	systolic ejection click
收缩期前奔马律	presystolic gallop
收缩期杂音	systolic murmur
收缩压	systolic pressure
收缩早期喀喇音	early systolic ejection click
收缩早期喷射音	early systolic ejection sound
收缩中晚期喀喇音	middle and late systolic click
手足徐动症	athetosis
瘦长型,无力型	asthenic type
输精管	vas deferens
输卵管	fallopian tube
舒张期杂音	diastolic murmur
舒张晚期奔马律	late diastolic gallop
舒张压	diastolic pressure
舒张早期奔马律	protodiastolic gallop
数目	number
双峰脉	bisferiens pulse
双手触诊法	bimanual palpation

水冲脉	water-hammer pulse
水坑试验	puddle test
水母头	caput medusa
水泡	vesicle
水泡音	bubble sound
水肿	edema
思维	thinking
四音律	quadruple rhythm
锁骨上窝	supraclavicular fossa
锁骨下窝	infraclavicular fossa
锁骨中线	midclavicular line

T

塔颅	tower skull
瘫痪	paralysis
弹性	elasticity
叹息样呼吸	sighing breath
特发性多发性斑状色素沉着	melanosis mecularis multiplex idiopathicum
提睾反射	cremasteric reflexes
提睾肌	cremaster
体表图形觉	graphesthesia
体格检查	physical examination
体位	position
体温	temperature
体型	habitus
体循环淤血	systemic congestion

体质性高身材	constitution tall stature
体重图	weight chart
体重指数	body mass index, BMI
调节	accommodation
听力	auditory acuity
听诊	auscultation
听诊器	stethoscope
通常分裂	general splitting
瞳孔	pupil
桶状胸	barrel chest
痛风石	tophus
痛性痉挛	cramps
头发	hair
头颅	skull
头皮	scalp
透光试验	transillumination
湍流	turbulent flow
脱肛	hedrocele
脱落脉	dropped pulse
托马斯征	Thomas sign
驼背	gibbus

W

蛙腹	frog belly
外耳道	external auditory canal
外形	contour
外展神经	abducent n.

往返性杂音	pro and to murmur
韦伯尔试验	Weber test, WT
萎黄病	chlorosis
胃泡鼓音区	Traube semilunar space
位听神经	auditory n.
胃型	gastral pattern
无害性杂音	innocent murmur, innocuous murmur
无力型(瘦长型)	asthenic type
无脉	pulseless
舞蹈样震颤	choreic movement

X

膝反射	patellar reflex
细湿啰音	fine rales
下腹部	hypogastric region
下疳	chancre
下肢压陷性水肿	peripheral pitting edema
消瘦	emaciation
小颅	microcephalia
小脑	cerebellum
斜颈	torticollis
心包积液	pericardial effusion
心包叩击音	pericardial knock
心包摩擦感	pericardial friction rub
心包摩擦音	pericardial friction sound
心动过缓	bradycardia

心动过速	tachycardia
心房颤动	atrial fibrillation
心肌肥厚	cardiomegaly, hypercardiotrophy
心尖搏动	apical impulse
心尖部（二尖瓣区）	mitral valve area
心力衰竭	heart failure
心律	cardiac rhythm
心率	heart rate
心率变异性	heart rate variability, HRV
心律失常	cardiac arrhythmia
心排血量降低	reduction in cardiac output
心前区隆起	protrusion of precordium
心室增大	ventricular hypertrophy
心音	cardiac sound
心音分裂	splitting of heart sound
心脏瓣膜听诊区	auscultatory valve area
心脏扩大	cardiac dilation
心脏损伤后综合征	Dressler's syndrome
心脏杂音	cardiac murmur
心脏增大	cardiac enlargement
心浊音界	cardiac dullness border
性别	sex
性腺发育不全（Turner 综合征）	gonadal dysgenesis
胸壁	chest wall

胸腹水	hydrothorax and ascites
胸骨柄	manubrium sterni
胸骨角	sterna angle
胸骨旁线	parasternal line
胸骨上切迹	suprasternal notch
胸骨上窝	suprasternal fossa
胸骨下角	infrasternal angle
胸骨线	sterna line
胸廓扩张度	thoracic expansion
胸膜壁层	parietal pleura
胸膜摩擦感	pleural friction fremitus
胸膜摩擦音	pleural friction rub
胸腔积液	pleural effusion
胸式呼吸	thoracic respiration
胸语音	pectoriloquy
嗅神经	olfactory n.
嗅诊	olfactory examination
漩涡	vortices
血色素沉着症	hematochromatosis
血压	blood pressure, BP
血肿	hematoma

Y

压痛	tenderness
压陷性水肿	pitting edema
牙齿	teeth
牙龈	gum

亚硝酸异戊酯试验	amyl nitrite test
颜面	face
眼睑	eyelids
眼内压	intraocular pressure, IOP
眼球	eyeball
眼球突出	exophthalmos
眼球下陷	enophthalmos
眼球震颤	nystagmus
羊鸣音	egophony
腰大肌试验	iliopsoas test
液波震颤	fluid wave thrills
腋后线	posterior axillary line
叶间隙	interlobar fissures
腋前线	anterior axillary line
腋窝	axillary fossa
腋中线	midaxillary line
一般状态	appearance
移动性浊音	shifting dullness
移行性舌炎	migratory glossitis
异常呼吸音	abnormal breath sounds
异常肌肉运动	abnormal muscle activities
意识模糊	confusion
意识障碍	disturbance of consciousness
意识状态	consciousness
意向性震颤	intentional tremor
阴道	vaginal
阴蒂	clitoris

阴阜	mons pubis
阴茎	penis
阴茎颈	neck of penis
阴茎头	glans penis
阴茎头冠	corona glandis
阴囊	scrotum
阴囊疝	scrotal hernia
阴囊湿疹	scrotal eczema
阴囊象皮病	scrotum elephantiasis
阴囊象皮肿	chyloderma
音叉试验	tuning fork test
隐睾症	cryptorchism
由蹲位到站立位	squatting to standing
硬度	consistency
右季肋部	right hypochondrial region
右髂部	right iliac region
右上腹部	right upper quadrant, RUQ
右下腹部	right lower quadrant, RLQ
右心衰竭	right-side heart failure
右腰部	right lumber region
瘀斑	ecchymosis
瘀点	petechia
语态	voice
语调	tone
语音共振	vocal resonance
语音震颤	vocal fremitus
原发性高血压,	essential hypertension

高血压病	
运动性失语	motor aphasia

Z

脏层胸膜	visceral pleura
谵妄	delirium
辗转体位	alternative position
张力障碍	dystonia
震颤	thrill, tremor
震颤麻痹	Parkinson's disease
震动觉	vibration
阵挛	clonus
振水音	succussion splash
正力型,匀称型	ortho-sthenic type
继发性高血压 症状性高血压,	secondary hypertension
肢端肥大症面容	acromegaly facies
肢端色素沉着症	acropigmentation
知觉	perception
知觉障碍	disturbance of perception
支气管肺泡呼吸音	bronchovesicular breath sound
支气管呼吸音	bronchial breath sound
支气管语音	bronchophony
蜘蛛痣	spider angioma
直肠脱垂	proctoptosis
直接叩诊	immediate percussion

直接叩诊法	direct percussion
直接听诊法	direct auscultation
直腿抬高加强试验	Lasegue sign
指鼻试验	finger nose test
指指试验	finger finger test
痔	hemorrhoid
智能	intelligence
中等	fairly
中腹部	umbilical region
中湿啰音	medium rales
肿瘤扑落音	tumor plop
重搏脉	dicrotic pulse
重点深入检查	focused examination
重点体格检查	problem-focused physical examination
舟状腹	scaphoid abdomen
主动脉瓣第二听诊区	the second aortic valve area
主动脉瓣关闭不全	aortic insufficiency, aortic regurgitation
主动脉瓣区	aortic valve area
主动脉瓣狭窄	aortic stenosis
主动脉喀喇音	aortic ejection click
注意	attention
浊音	dullness
姿势	posture
姿势性震颤	postural tremor

紫癜	purpura
子宫附件	uterine adnexa
自主体位	active position
醉酒步态	drinken man gait
左季肋部	left hypochondrial region
左髂部	left iliac region
左上腹部	left upper quadrant, LUQ
左下腹部	left lower quadrant, LLQ
左心衰竭	left-side heart failure
左腰部	left lumber region
坐位屈颈试验	Lindner test

徐蓓莉(Xu Beili)　石虹(Shi Hong)

附录4 《临床诊断学》英文—中文单词表

(按英文字母顺序)

A

abdominal concavity	腹部凹陷
abdominal mass	腹部肿块
abdominal protuberance	腹部膨隆
abdominal reflexes	腹壁反射
abducent n.	外展神经
abnormal breath sounds	异常呼吸音
abnormal movements	不自主运动
abnormal muscle activities	异常肌肉运动
acanthosis nigricans	黑棘皮病
accommodation	调节
achilles reflex	跟腱反射
acro-cephalosyndactylia	尖颅并指(趾)畸形
acromegaly facies	肢端肥大症面容
acropachy	杵状指(趾)
acropigmentation	肢端色素沉着症
active position	自主体位
Addison disease	艾迪生病,肾上腺皮质功能减退症

adventitious sound	附加音
affect	情感反应
after depolarization	后除极
age	年龄
agraphia	失写症
air conduction	气导
albinismus	白化病
alexia	失读症
alternate motion	轮替动作
alternative position	辗转体位
ambulatory blood pressure measurement, ABPM	动态血压监测
amphorophony	空瓮音
amyl nitrite test	亚硝酸异戊酯试验
anal canal	肛管
anal fissure	肛裂
ankle clonus	踝阵挛
anterior axillary line	腋前线
anterior midline	前正中线
anterior superior iliac spine	髂前上棘
aortic ejection click	主动脉喀喇音
aortic insufficiency	主动脉瓣关闭不全
aortic regurgitation	主动脉瓣关闭不全
aortic stenosis	主动脉瓣狭窄
aortic valve area	主动脉瓣区
aphasia	失语
apical belly	尖腹

apical impulse	心尖搏动
appearance	一般状态
apraxia	失用症
arcus senilis	老年环
areola of breast	乳晕
arm circumference	上臂周径
ascites	腹水
asthenic type	瘦长型,无力型
ataxia	共济失调
ataxic gait	共济失调步态
atelectasis	肺不张
athetosis	手足徐动症
atrial fibrillation	心房颤动
atrial gallop	房性奔马律
attention	注意
auditory acuity	听力
auditory n.	位听神经
auricle	耳廓
auscultation	听诊
auscultatory valve area	心脏瓣膜听诊区
axillary fossa	腋窝

B

Babinski's sign	巴彬斯基征
ballottement	冲击触诊法
barrel chest	桶状胸
basal ganglion	基底节

beefy tongue	牛肉舌
biceps reflex	肱二头肌反射
bigeminal beats	二联律
bimanual palpation	双手触诊法
bisferiens pulse	双峰脉
bleb	疱疹
blood pressure, BP	血压
board-like rigidity	板状腹
body mass index, BMI	体重指数
bone conduction	骨导
bowel sound	肠鸣音
bradycardia	心动过缓
bradypnea	呼吸过缓
breast	乳房
breathing movement	呼吸运动
bronchial breath sound	支气管呼吸音
bronchophony	支气管语音
bronchovesicular breath sound	支气管肺泡呼吸音
Brudzinski's sign	布鲁津斯基征
bubble sound	水泡音

C

cachexia	恶病质
cannon wave, cannon "a" wave	巨大 a 波
capillary pulsation sign	毛细血管搏动征

caput medusa	水母头
cardiac arrhythmia	心律失常
cardiac dilation	心脏扩大
cardiac dullness border	心浊音界
cardiac enlargement	心脏增大
cardiac murmur	心脏杂音
cardiac rhythm	心律
cardiac sound	心音
cardiomegaly	心肌肥厚
carotene	胡萝卜素
cerebellum	小脑
cervix uteri	宫颈
Chaddock's sign	查多克征
chancre	下疳
chancroid	软下疳
chest wall	胸壁
Cheyne-Stokes breathing	潮式呼吸
chloasma	黄褐斑
chlorosis	萎黄病
choreic movement	舞蹈样震颤
chyloderma	阴囊象皮肿
clitoris	阴蒂
clonus	阵挛
coarse rales	粗湿啰音
cochlear n.	耳蜗神经
color sensation	色觉
coma	昏迷

complete physical examination	全身体格检查
compulsive position	强迫体位
compulsive squatting	强迫蹲位
confusion	意识模糊
conjunctiva	结膜
consciousness	意识状态
consistency	硬度
consolidation of lung	肺实变
constitution tall stature	体质性高身材
continuous murmur	连续性杂音
contour	外形
convergency reflex	集合反射
cornea	角膜
corneal reflex	角膜反射
corona glandis	阴茎头冠
corpus uteri	宫体
costal margin	肋弓下缘
costovertebral angle	肋脊角
Courvoisier sign	库瓦洛埃征
crackle	爆裂音
cramps	痛性痉挛
cranial n.	脑神经
cremaster	提睾肌
cremasteric reflexes	提睾反射
crepitus	捻发音
cretinism	呆小病

critical facies	病危面容
cryptorchism	隐睾症
Cushing syndrome	库欣综合征
cutaneous hemangiomas	皮肤血管瘤
cyanosis	发绀
cycled respiration test	深呼吸试验

D

deafness	耳聋
deep palpation	深部触诊法
deep press palpation	深压触诊法
deep slipping palpation	深部滑行触诊法
deforming skull	变形颅
delichocephalia	长颅
delirium	谵妄
dementia	痴呆
deMusset's sign	点头运动
desquamation	皮肤脱屑
development	发育
diaphragmatic respiration	腹式呼吸
diastolic murmur	舒张期杂音
diastolic pressure	舒张压
dicrotic pulse	重搏脉
diplopia	复视
direct auscultation	直接听诊法
direct percussion	直接叩诊法
disorders of sensation	感觉障碍

disorientation	定向障碍
disturbance of consciousness	意识障碍
disturbance of perception	知觉障碍
Gordon's sign	戈登征
dough kneading sensation	揉面感
Dressler's syndrome	心脏损伤后综合征
drinken man gait	醉酒步态
dropped pulse	脱落脉
dry rales	干啰音
Dugas' sign	杜加斯征
dullness	浊音
Duroziez's sign	杜柔双重音
dysphonia	构音困难
dyspnea	呼吸困难
dystonia	张力障碍

E

early systolic ejection click	收缩早期喀喇音
early systolic ejection sound	收缩早期喷射音
ecchymosis	瘀斑
edema	水肿
egophony	羊鸣音
ejection sound	喷射音
elasticity	弹性
ely test	跟臀试验
emaciation	消瘦

emotion	情感
enophthalmos	眼球下陷
entropion	睑内翻
epididymal cyst	附睾囊肿
epididymis	附睾
epigastric region	上腹部
epistaxis	鼻出血
erection	勃起
erosion	糜烂
erythema nodosum	结节性红斑
essential hypertension	原发性高血压,高血压病
exophthalmos	眼球突出
expression	表情
external auditory canal	外耳道
extra cardiac sound	额外心音
eyeball	眼球
eyelids	眼睑

F

face	颜面
facial features	面容
facial n.	面神经
fairly	中等
fallopian tube	输卵管
familial progressive hyperpigmantation	家族性进行性色素过度沉着症

fasciculation	肌束颤动
festinating gait	慌张步态
fine rales	细湿啰音
finger finger test	指指试验
finger nose test	指鼻试验
first heart sound	第一心音
fixed splitting	固定分裂
flat chest	扁平胸
flatness	实音
fluctuation	波动感
fluid wave thrills	液波震颤
focused examination	重点深入检查
forced standing position	强迫停立位
fourth heart sound	第四心音
freckle	雀斑
free ribs	浮肋
friction rubs	摩擦音
frog belly	蛙腹
functional murmur	功能性杂音
funnel chest	漏斗胸

G

gait	步态
gallop rhythm	奔马律
gastral pattern	胃型
general splitting	通常分裂
geographic tongue	地图舌

Gibson murmur	机器声样杂音
gibbus	驼背
glans penis	阴茎头
glossopharyngeal n.	舌咽神经
gonadal dysgenesis	性腺发育不全（Turner 综合征）
graphesthesia	体表图形觉
gum	牙龈
gurgling sound	咕噜声

H

habitus	体型
hair	头发,毛发
hairy tongue	毛舌
hallucination	幻觉
Harrison's groove	肋膈沟
heart failure	心力衰竭
heart rate	心率
heart rate variability, HRV	心率变异性
hedrocele	脱肛
heel jar test	后跟试验
heel-knee-tibia test	跟膝胫试验
hematoma	血肿
hematochromatosis	血色素沉着症
hemorrhoid	痔
hepatic facies	肝病面容
hepatojugular reflux	肝颈静脉回流

hepatolenticular degeneration	肝豆状核变性
hepatomegaly	肝大
hoarseness	声嘶
Hoffmann's sign	霍夫曼征
holosystolic murmur	全收缩期杂音
hook method	钩指触诊法
hook technique	钩指触诊
hydrocele of cord	精索积液
hydrothorax and ascites	胸腹水
hymen	处女膜
hypercardiotrophy	心肌肥厚
hyperesthesia	感觉过敏
hyperkeratosis of the nipple and areola	乳头乳晕角化过度症
hyperresonance	过清音
hypertension	高血压
hyperthyroidism	甲状腺功能亢进
hypoesthesia	感觉减退
hypogastric region	下腹部
hypoglossal n.	舌下神经
hypotension	低血压

I

ideal body weight	理想体重
iliopsoas test	腰大肌试验
illusion	错觉

immediate percussion	直接叩诊
indirect auscultation	间接听诊法
indirect percussion	间接叩诊法
infraclavicular fossa	锁骨下窝
infrascapular region	肩胛下区
infrasternal angle	胸骨下角
inguinal ligament	腹股沟韧带
innocent murmur, innocuous murmur	无害性杂音
inspection	视诊
intelligence	智能
intentional tremor	意向性震颤
intercostal space	肋间隙
interlobar fissures	叶间隙
intermittent claudication	间歇性跛行
interscapular region	肩胛间区
intestinal pattern	肠型
intraocular pressure, IOP	眼内压
inward impulse	负性心尖搏动
iris	虹膜
isometric hand grip	等张握力运动

J

jaundice	黄疸
joint position sense	关节觉
jugular vein distension	颈静脉充盈

K

keeled chest	鸡胸
Kernig's sign	凯尔尼格征
Klinefelter syndrome	克莱恩费特综合征
koilonychia	匙状指
Koplik spot	麻疹黏膜斑
kyphosis	脊柱后凸

L

labium majus	大阴唇
laminar flow	层流
large skull	巨颅
laryngeal pharynx	喉咽
larynx	喉
Lasegue sign	直腿抬高加强试验
late diastolic gallop	舒张晚期奔马律
lateral border of rectus muscles	腹直肌外缘
left hypochondrial region	左季肋部
left iliac region	左髂部
left lower quadrant, LLQ	左下腹部
left lumber region	左腰部
left upper quadrant, LUQ	左上腹部
left-side heart failure	左心衰竭
lentigo simplex	单纯雀斑样痣
leukoplakia	白斑

light palpation	浅部触诊法
Lindner test	坐位屈颈试验
linea alba	腹白线
liver thrill	肝震颤
location	部位
lordosis	脊柱前凸

M

machinery murmur	机器声样杂音
maculae	斑疹
maculopapular	斑丘疹
major vestibular grands	前庭大腺
malignant melanoma	恶性黑色素瘤
manubrium sterni	胸骨柄
mass	包块
mastoid	乳突
McBurney point	麦氏点,阑尾点
mediate percussion	间接叩诊
medium rales	中湿啰音
melanin	黑色素
melanosis mecularis multiplex idiopathicum	特发性多发性斑状色素沉着
memory	记忆
mental disorder	精神障碍
mental status	精神状态
microcephalia	小颅
midabdominal line	腹中线

midaxillary line	腋中线
midclavicular line	锁骨中线
middle and late systolic click	收缩中晚期喀喇音
migratory glossitis	移行性舌炎
mitral facies	二尖瓣面容
mitral insufficiency	二尖瓣关闭不全
mitral regurgitation	二尖瓣反流
mitral stenosis	二尖瓣狭窄
mitral valve area	心尖部(二尖瓣区)
mitral valve prolapse syndrome	二尖瓣脱垂综合征
mobility	活动度
moist rale	湿啰音
moisture	湿度
Mongolian spot	蒙古斑
mons pubis	阴阜
moon facies	满月面容
motor aphasia	运动性失语
mouth	口
muscle tone	肌张力
myoclonus	肌阵挛
myokymia	肌纤维颤搐
myxedema	黏液性水肿

N

nasal pharynx	鼻咽

nasal sinus	鼻窦
near reflex	近反射
neck of penis	阴茎颈
nephritic facies	肾病面容
nipple	乳头
nominal aphasia	命名性失语
number	数目
nystagmus	眼球震颤

O

obesity	肥胖
obturator maneuver	闭孔内肌试验
oculomotor n.	动眼神经
olfactory examination	嗅诊
olfactory n.	嗅神经
opening snap	开瓣音
ophthalmoscope	检眼镜
opisthotonos position	角弓反张位
Oppenheim's sign	奥本海姆征
oppositional paratonia	抵抗
optic n.	视神经
oral pharynx	口咽
orange peel	橘皮
organic murmur	器质性杂音
orientation	定向力
orthopnea	端坐呼吸
ortho-sthenic type	正力型,匀称型

ovary	卵巢
oxycephaly	尖颅

P

pallor	苍白
palpation	触诊
pansystolic murmur	全收缩期杂音
papules	丘疹
paradoxical pulse, pulsus paradoxus	奇脉
paradoxical splitting	反常分裂
paralysis	瘫痪
paralytic squint	麻痹性斜视
parasternal line	胸骨旁线
parietal pleura	胸膜壁层
Parkinson's disease	震颤麻痹
parotid gland	腮腺
passive leg raising maneuver	被动抬腿动作
passive position	被动体位
patella clonus	髌阵挛
patellar	膝反射
pectoriloquy	胸语音
penis	阴茎
perception	知觉
percussion	叩诊
percussion sound	叩诊音

pericardial effusion	心包积液
pericardial friction sound	心包摩擦音
pericardial knock	心包叩击音
pericardium friction rub	心包摩擦感
perineum	会阴
peripheral pitting edema	下肢压陷性水肿
peristalsis	蠕动波
peritoneal irritation sign	腹膜刺激征
petechia	瘀点
Peutz Jeghers syndrome	色素沉着-息肉综合征
phimosis	包茎
physical examination	体格检查
physiologic splitting	生理性分裂
pigeon chest	鸡胸
pigmentation	色素沉着
pistol shot	枪击音
pitting edema	压陷性水肿
pleural effusion	胸腔积液
pleural friction fremitus	胸膜摩擦感
pleural friction rub	胸膜摩擦音
pneumoperitoneum	气腹
pneumothorax	气胸
poorly	不良
position	体位
posterior axillary line	腋后线
posterior midline	后正中线

postural tremor	姿势性震颤
posture	姿势
premature contraction	期前收缩
prepuce	包皮
prepuce redundant	包皮过长
presystolic gallop	收缩期前奔马律
pro and to murmur	往返性杂音
problem-focused physical examination	重点体格检查
proctoptosis	直肠脱垂
prostate gland	前列腺
protodiastolic gallop	舒张早期奔马律
protrusion of precordium	心前区隆起
psychosensory disturbance	感知综合障碍
ptosis	上睑下垂
puddle test	水坑试验
pulmonary congestion	肺循环淤血
pulmonary ejection click	肺动脉喀喇音
pulmonary emphysema	肺气肿
pulmonary valve area	肺动脉瓣区
pulsation of carotid artery	颈动脉搏动
pulse	脉搏
pulse deficit	脉搏短绌,短绌脉
pulse pressure, PP	脉压
pulseless	无脉
pulsus alternans	交替脉
pupil	瞳孔

purpura	紫癜
pustule	脓疱

Q

quadruple rhythm	四音律

R

rachitic chest	佝偻病胸
rachitic rosary	佝偻病串珠
radial periosteal	桡反射
rales	啰音
rebound tenderness	反跳痛
redness	发红
reduction in cardiac output	心排血量降低
referred pain	牵涉痛
referred tenderness	牵涉性触痛
reflex	发射
resonance	清音
respiration	呼吸
respiratory depth	呼吸深度
respiratory frequency	呼吸频率
respiratory rhythm and range	呼吸节律和幅度
reversed splitting	逆分裂
rib	肋骨
right hypochondrial region	右季肋部
right iliac region	右髂部

right lower quadrant, RLQ	右下腹部
right lumber region	右腰部
right upper quadrant, RUQ	右上腹部
right-side heart failure	右心衰竭
Rinne test, RT	任内试验
rhonchi	干啰音
Romberg's sign	昂白征
rosacea	酒渣鼻
roseola	玫瑰疹
Rovsing's test	结肠充气试验
ruler pressing test	尺压试验

S

saddle nose	鞍鼻
sardonic feature	苦笑面容
scalp	头皮
scaphoid abdomen	舟状腹
scapular line	肩胛线
scapular region	肩胛区
scapula	肩胛骨
scar	瘢痕
Schwabach test, ST	施瓦巴赫试验
scissors gait	剪刀式步态
sclera	巩膜
scoliosis	脊柱侧凸
scratch test	搔刮试验
screening examination	筛查

scrotal eczema	阴囊湿疹
scrotal hernia	阴囊疝
scrotum	阴囊
scrotum elephantiasis	阴囊象皮病
second heart sound	第二心音
secondary hypertension	继发性高血压,症状性高血压
seminal vesicle	精囊
sensation	感觉
sensory aphasia	感觉性失语
setting sun phenomenon	落日现象
sex	性别
shifting dullness	移动性浊音
sibilant rhonchi	高调干啰音
sighing breath	叹息样呼吸
sinus phrenicocostalis	肋膈窦
size	大小
skin eruption	皮疹
skinfold thickness	皮褶厚度
skull	头颅
smegma	包皮垢
smooth tongue	光滑舌
somnolence	嗜睡
sonorous rhonchi	低调干啰音
spasm	痉挛
spermatic cord	精索
spermatocele	精子囊肿

spider angioma	蜘蛛痣
spinal accessory n.	副神经
spinous process	脊柱棘突
splenomegaly	脾大
splitting of heart sound	心音分裂
squared skull	方颅
squatting to standing	由蹲位到站立位
stained yellow	黄染
static tremor	静止性震颤
steppage gait	跨阈步态
stereognosis	实体辨别觉
sterna angle	胸骨角
sterna line	胸骨线
stethoscope	听诊器
sthenic type	超力型,矮胖型
strawberry tongue	草莓舌
stupor	昏睡
subcutaneous bleeding	皮下出血
subcutaneous emphysema	皮下气肿
subcutaneous nodules	皮下结节
succussion splash	振水音
summation gallop	重叠性奔马律
supraclavicular fossa	锁骨上窝
suprascapular region	肩胛上区
suprasternal fossa	胸骨上窝
suprasternal notch	胸骨上切迹
symmetry	对称性

systemic congestion	体循环淤血
systolic ejection click	收缩期喀喇音
systolic murmur	收缩期杂音
systolic pressure	收缩压

T

tachycardia	心动过速
tachypnea	呼吸过速
tactile fremitus	触觉震颤
tardus pulse	迟脉
teeth	牙齿
temperature	体温
tenderness	压痛
testis	睾丸
the second aortic valve area	主动脉瓣第二听诊区
third heart sound	第三心音
Thomas sign	托马斯征
thoracic expansion	胸廓扩张度
thoracic respiration	胸式呼吸
three depressions sign	三凹征
thrill	震颤
thyroid	甲状腺
tics	抽搐
tidal breathing	潮式呼吸
tone	语调
tongue	舌
tophus	痛风石

torticollis	斜颈
tower skull	塔颅
transient arterial occlusion	短暂阻断动脉血流
transillumination	透光试验
traube semilunar space	胃泡鼓音区
tremor	震颤
Trendelenburg test	髋关节承重功能试验
triceps reflex	肱三头肌反射
tricuspid valve area	三尖瓣区
trigeminal beats	三联律
trigeminal n.	三叉神经
triggered activity	触发活动
trochlear n.	滑车神经
tumor plop	肿瘤扑落音
tuning fork test	音叉试验
turbulent flow	湍流
two-point tactile discrimination	两点辨别感觉
tympany	鼓音
typhoid facies	伤寒面容

U

ulcer	溃疡
umbilical region	脐部,中腹部
umbilicus	脐
upper abdominal angle	腹上角
urethral meatus	尿道口

urticaria	荨麻疹
uterine adnexa	子宫附件
uterus	子宫

V

vaginal	阴道
vagus n.	迷走神经
Valsalva maneuver	Valsalva 动作
vas deferens	输精管
vein	静脉
ventricular gallop	室性奔马律
ventricular hypertrophy	心室增大
vesicle	水泡
vesicular breath sound	肺泡呼吸音
vestibular nerve	前庭神经
vibration	震动觉
visceral pleura	脏层胸膜
visual acuity	视力
visual disorder	视力障碍
visual fields	视野
vital sign	生命征
vitiligo	白癜
vocal fremitus	语音震颤
vocal resonance	语音共振
voice	语态
vortices	漩涡

W

waddling gait	蹒跚步态
water-hammer pulse	水冲脉
Weber test, WT	韦伯尔试验
weight chart	体重图
whispered pectoriloquy	耳语音增强
Wright-Schober test	瑞-舒测试法
wrinkled tongue	裂纹舌

X

xiphoid process	剑突

徐蓓莉(Xu Beili)　石虹(Shi Hong)

图书在版编目(CIP)数据

规范体格检查与病史书写双语手册/傅志君,石虹主编.—上海:复旦大学出版社,2009.6(2020.9重印)
ISBN 978-7-309-06554-1

Ⅰ.规… Ⅱ.①傅…②石… Ⅲ.病案-书写规划-手册-英、汉
Ⅳ.R197.323-62

中国版本图书馆 CIP 数据核字(2009)第 040476 号

规范体格检查与病史书写双语手册
傅志君　石　虹　主编
责任编辑/肖　英

复旦大学出版社有限公司出版发行
上海市国权路 579 号　邮编:200433
网址: fupnet@ fudanpress.com　http://www.fudanpress.com
门市零售:86-21-65102580　团体订购:86-21-65104505
外埠邮购:86-21-65642846　出版部电话:86-21-65642845
浙江临安曙光印务有限公司

开本 787×960　1/32　印张 5.625　字数 97 千
2020 年 9 月第 1 版第 4 次印刷

ISBN 978-7-309-06554-1/R·1078
定价:15.00 元

如有印装质量问题,请向复旦大学出版社出版部调换。
版权所有　　侵权必究